"My Kid's Allergic to Everything"
Dessert Cookbook

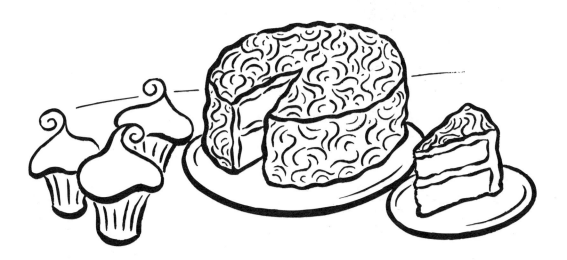

Mary Harris and Wilma Nachsin

Forewords by
Dr. Rebecca Hoffman and Dr. Ida Mary S. Thoma

CHICAGO
REVIEW
PRESS

Library of Congress Cataloging-in-Publication Data

Harris, Mary, 1953–
    My kid's allergic to everything dessert cookbook: sweets and treats the whole family will enjoy/
Mary Harris and Wilma Nachsin; forewords by Rebecca Hoffman and Ida Mary S. Thoma.
        p.   cm.
    Includes index.
    ISBN 1-55652-303-3
    1. Food allergy in children—Diet therapy—Recipes. 2. Desserts. I. Nachsin, Wilma, 1954–. II. Title.
RJ386.5.H37 1996
618.92'9750654—dc20   96-42047
                                                                                                          CIP

© 1996 by Mary Harris and Wilma Nachsin
Illustrated by Rita Daugavietis
First edition
Published by Chicago Review Press, Incorporated
814 North Franklin Street
Chicago, Illinois 60610
ISBN 1-55652-303-3
Printed in the United States of America
5 4 3 2 1

Contents

Foreword

Dr. Rebecca S. Hoffman

When I was asked to write a foreword for this cookbook, I was pleased that another resource would be available to help my patients with food allergies. As we all know, adhering to special dietary constraints is very difficult, especially for children. This cookbook will broaden the menu choices available and provide some inspiration for developing many new recipe alternatives.

Food allergies manifest themselves in many ways: skin rashes such as eczema, nasal congestion, runny nose, frequent upper respiratory infections, hives, headaches, asthma, even life-threatening anaphylaxis.

Infants and very young children with allergies are often sensitive to foods, the most common sensitivities being to eggs, milk, wheat, soy, corn, and peanuts. Children and adults may also have additional reactions to inhalant allergens such as dust mites, molds, pollens, and animal danders.

One clue to look for when you think someone in your family has food allergies is an itchy, red, scaly skin rash, especially on the face or neck, or inside the elbows or behind the knees, that persists for weeks or months and may wax and wane over time. The rash may flare up after the individual eats a particular food, but sometimes this is too subtle to see. Another clinical sign of allergies in general is a cold that won't go away—runny, stuffy nose, cough, and fatigue. Asthma can also be a problem; this can be manifested by coughing, wheezing, shortness of breath, or a tight or congested chest. These symptoms occur either in a seasonal pattern or after exposure to a specific allergen such as a cat, exposure to a cold, or exercise.

Food allergy-induced asthma can also be part of the syndrome of anaphylaxis, which is a severe and sudden allergic reaction resulting in multiple symptoms such as hives, low blood pressure, difficulty breathing, and abdominal cramping and diarrhea. Food anaphylaxis is a life-threatening type of food allergy.

As you can see, food and inhalant allergies can show up in many different ways. The first step is to be suspicious of an allergy, either because of the nature of the symptoms or because of a family history of allergies. Next you should look carefully at the possible allergens: foods, dust, dander, etc. Then work with your pediatrician, internist, family practitioner, or allergist to identify the problem areas. A good history of the symptoms, a complete physical examination, and a few selected tests should pinpoint the most likely offending allergens. Finally, working with your physician through elimination of foods and/or decreasing exposure to other environmental allergens should help toward eliminating chronic symptoms. For food allergies, elimination of the offending items is the only current proven method of symptom relief. Sometimes, this is very difficult to accomplish, especially if the allergy is to something as all-pervasive as wheat or eggs. That is where this book offers hope and practical help.

The one good thing about food allergies is that, with strict avoidance, some children will eventually lose their sensitivity to a food. However, some food allergies do persist for life. Depending on the severity of the original reactions, repeat testing and even controlled food challenges can be done periodically to test for continued allergies.

Knowledge about the problem and perseverance in its treatment can usually control food and other allergies relatively well. As of yet, there is no cure for allergies, but with continued research, we may hope for medical breakthroughs.

Foreword

Dr. Ida Mary S. Thoma

How wonderful for a child to have tasty snacks and fun foods without itching or wheezing! A happy stress-free person (child or adult) is more apt to "outgrow" allergic manifestations. I wish that I had just such a cookbook as this one when I was dealing with food allergies in my family.

I have found through personal and family experiences that food allergies may cause a variety of symptoms. In our family, the hives and eczema (atopic dermatitis) suffered by one of our children was suspected to be caused by a food allergy. Our family doctor, S. C. Lavine, initially sent us to a dermatologist who chose to treat only the symptoms. Knowing of my background in immunology, Dr. Lavine then suggested that I track down the offending allergens, those foods that caused the dermatitis.

As eliminating one food at a time did not alleviate the symptoms, we knew that more than one food was involved. We then resorted to the following method, which I recommend be used under your doctor's guidance and with his or her approval:

1. Keep a food diary.

2. After one week of listing all foods eaten, eliminate completely a selected food that has been eaten daily from the diet for four or five days. For example, if wheat is the test food, eliminate all wheat in any form.

3. On the fourth or fifth day at breakfast (or at least eight hours after any other foods have been ingested), the test food only, in its purest form, should be eaten, e.g., cream of wheat cereal, seasoned with salt only.

4. The person being tested should be observed for allergic reactions. If the food is indeed an allergen, within 15 to 30 minutes one or more symptoms may occur: itching; a burning sensation; chills; a headache or an aura of bright lights or spots before the eyes; swelling of the nasal passages; wheezing; perhaps, within an hour or so, diarrhea. If no symptoms occur, there is no strong allergy to the test food. We have found that if there is a strong allergic reaction, a dose of milk of magnesia will hasten the riddance of the allergen from the body.

To summarize the procedure that was successful for us:

1. The test food must be eaten daily for one week before the test.

2. The test food must then be eliminated completely from the diet for four or five days.

3. The test food alone must be given to the subject after he or she has fasted for at least eight hours. A single food is tested at one time. I allowed 24 hours or longer between tests, and tested only at breakfast.

4. The person must be observed carefully for at least 40 to 60 minutes after ingesting the food.

In this way I found that our daughter was allergic to corn, oatmeal, and lamb (including lanolin in hand creams, as well as wool).

The food diary was extremely important. I used one page in a loose-leaf notebook to record for one week the foods eaten at each meal, as well as extra snacks and drinks ingested between meals. All changes, good or bad, in the general well-being of the allergic person were noted in the diary. The food diary also serves as a menu planner—useful in spacing foods to prevent the allergic person from developing additional food allergies. Additional food allergies sometimes develop when one food or another is eaten frequently over a long period of time. If the daily menu is varied and a particular food is given only every four or five days, there seems to be no increase in allergies. I think this is especially true of infants who show allergic reactions. Some of the more common allergens that it is wise to "space" are wheat and wheat products, corn and corn products, chocolate, oranges, oatmeal, eggs and egg products, and peanut butter. To avoid identified allergens, it is important to read all labels carefully on all containers of prepared or processed foods, including canned and frozen foods, confections and snack foods, mixes, drinks, breads and cakes, salad dressings, and preserves.

In order to have a varied menu and still eliminate identified allergens, I found it necessary to prepare meals from simple, pure, basic ingredients, free of the substances causing the allergies, instead of the many foods we had been buying in processed forms. That is why I am so appreciative of this cookbook and all the possibilities for fun foods that it offers.

Acknowledgments

We wish to thank Dr. Rebecca Hoffman and Dr. Ida Mary S. Thoma for their invaluable assistance in clarifying the medical aspects of asthma and allergies and their symptoms, for discussing the efficacy of a food elimination diet, and for their encouragement in our search for alternative foods and recipes. We also wish to thank Dr. David G. Fisher for his careful editing of the chapters regarding yeast and the family and species of alternative flours; and for providing an excellent appendix for those who wish to pursue the definitive origins of their ingredients. Our heartfelt thanks to our editor Cynthia Sherry for all her hard work and painstaking attention to detail. Thanks to Jim Morris for coming up with the perfect title. And most important, we thank Aaron, Jacob, Josh, Jessie, Andy, and Jonathan for their patience and their overworked tastebuds!

Introduction

This cookbook is designed for parents and caregivers who are coping with food allergies in their youngsters. You have picked up this book and started reading because you suspect, or your doctor has just told you, that your child is allergic to certain foods. You have noticed dark circles under your child's eyes, even after a good night's sleep; a wheezy sound when your child is breathing normally; a chronic stuffy or itchy nose; too many ear infections to be considered normal; dry, sensitive skin; a chronic cough when your child does not have a cold. As with any medical problem, you are urged to see your pediatrician if you haven't already; these symptoms are indications of allergies and asthma. However, if you feel your questions are not being addressed completely, *don't give up*! Continue talking to friends, reading health and nutrition literature, and looking for a doctor who will work with you and your child.

You, like us, want to be able to feed your child nutritious and healthy snacks that do not contain the foods he or she is allergic to. You want your child to be a normal part of the crowd and not to feel singled out by what he or she eats.

Our children have been coping with allergies to cow's milk, wheat, corn, peanuts, almonds, white potatoes, gluten, chocolate, and egg albumin (egg white) for many years. We searched health food stores, libraries, and bookstores for alternative recipes for our children's main meals, snacks, and special occasions. Because so many of the allergy books and cookbooks we reviewed contained mostly main course recipes for adults with allergies, we wanted to create a cookbook of special desserts and snacks especially for children. It's heartbreaking to see your child at a birthday party unable to eat the cake because it was made with bleached, enriched flour made from wheat, eggs, and commercial baking powder. It's difficult for children to understand that when they go to another child's birthday party they can't have the ice cream because it was made with cow's milk, eggs, and corn syrup sweeteners. It's hard to explain that they can't eat the candy, cookies, or potato chips on grocery shelves. We wanted to be able to provide as normal and healthy a diet as possible within their limitations.

We have created cake, pie, and cookie recipes for you to use on special occasions or just for fun. With our children's diet limitations, fun can be hard to find in the kitchen, and we believe childhood should be *fun*, not just healthy! We have also included a few breakfast ideas, modified for elimination diets.

In each recipe's list of ingredients, we have put the ingredient that works best first, e.g., 1½ cups oat flour *or* spelt flour *or* amaranth flour. This means we have achieved the tastiest results with oat flour, but have also been successful using the other flours. If there is only one ingredient listed in a line, this means we have not found (or do not need) any alternatives. Please feel free to substitute ingredients you find exciting to work with or that your child especially likes. Our recipes show our favorite way to achieve each result, but certainly not the only way! Please be aware, however, that flour and grain substitutions don't always work out well; trial and error is the only way for you to determine how to make your own substitutions.

It can be difficult to buy healthful snacks while traveling. We found acceptable snacks and ingredients not only at health food stores but also at local supermarkets, and we discuss those in chapter 10. Food allergies are often present with other allergies, asthma, and a wide variety of other health problems. We feel that the allergic reactions our children suffer from may be eased by eliminating many commercial chemical cleaners in our homes, by using products recommended by our doctors, and by using ecological pesticides and herbicides in our homes and gardens. While we are unaware of any medical studies to support this conclusion, we feel that the cleaner and safer the environment is, the easier it may be for children to cope with and outgrow their allergies, asthma, and other medical difficulties. Therefore, we have included some cleaning and pesticide tips and addresses of organizations that can provide more detailed information than we are able to include here; you may find other resources in ecology handbooks and your local newspaper.

If you are interested in trying to keep your home and garden as chemical-free as possible, we have also included sources for further information and suppliers for gardening and cleaning products.

Finally, we include a list of cookbooks that we found useful as starting points in our search for allergen-free recipes. We realize that alternative ingredients may be difficult to find in some areas, so we have included addresses for mail-order products. The inclusion of brand-name products, organizations, and manufacturers is not an endorsement of them by us, but rather a guide for you to use in searching out healthy alternative products. We have tried to verify that the manufacturers listed in the resources chapter can provide mail-order ingredients to individual consumers at a reasonable cost, and if they are organic that they can provide sufficient proof of their certification to the consumer. You may already have sources for special ingredients: if they are different from the ones listed here we would love to hear about them! Support organizations are also included if you would like to seek further information about your child's specific allergy, want to investigate further the possibility of creating a cleaner environment, or just want someone to talk with.

This cookbook is not intended to take the place of medical diagnosis or a nutritionist's services. It is intended only as a guide and resource for alternative ingredients and recipes. The publishers, authors, and contributors take no responsibility for this book's use as a substitute for qualified medical and nutritional diagnosis or for a consumer's unhappiness with a particular product. We have accepted no remuneration in any form from any of the companies listed herein.

1

Know Your Flours and Their Alter Egos

*U*sing alternative flours can be very confusing and scary. We live in a world full of prepackaged box mixes for pancakes, cakes, and muffins—when we were faced with using alternative flours and ingredients, we were thrown for a loop. What can be used in place of bleached, enriched flour made from wheat for a birthday cake? After the initial panic died down, we realized that there are many grains and flours that are just as easy to use as wheat, but the slightly different qualities, such as lower or absent gluten content, made finding the right proportions difficult. We explored many helpful resources, such as the University of Wisconsin's and the University of Illinois's extension offices, diet books, and health food stores' employees, but in the long run the best teacher was experience. A chart near the end of this chapter provides general information about using and combining these alternative flours. However, certain flours work better than others when preparing a variety of baked goods. For your convenience, specific combination charts listing flours that work best for each category of baked goods appear in chapters 3 through 7.

If you are dealing with a gluten allergy, a yeast allergy, or celiac disease (an allergy to proteins in many grains), most of the flours and recipes in this book will not work for you. Nongluten baked goods are extremely difficult to produce. Consequently, most of our recipes call for gluten flours.

Gluten is the elastic component in many grains that reacts with liquids and yeast in the unbaked dough, expanding and forming a network of tiny expandable pockets that trap the carbon dioxide created during the leavening process, thus making the dough "rise." Because wheat gluten is the stickiest and the most elastic of all grain glutens, it sets the standard for ease of preparation and rising in breads and other baked goods.

Yeast is a fungus that produces the carbon dioxide during fermentation. It continually reproduces itself, feeding off gluten and sugars.

Gluten and yeast, singly or together, give baked products their lighter texture and weight. Nongluten flours do not feed yeast at all; therefore "rising" must be forced either by adding a gluten flour to the nongluten flour in the recipe or by using a lot more of a different leavening agent, such as baking powder or baking soda with an acidic ingredient.

Wheat (and corn) flour is used in many products under many different names. When a label indicates that "modified food starch" or a "thickening agent" has been used, you may assume that wheat (or corn) in some form has been added. Surprisingly, even some candies, such as licorice, use wheat flour as a thickener and stiffener. Other ingredient and trademark names for wheat include bran, bread crumbs, bulgur or burghol, couscous, cracker meal, durum, farina, many forms of "filler," gluten, graham, HVP (hydrolyzed vegetable protein), many types of modified food starch, MSG, orzo, pumpernickel, seitan, semolina, tabbouleh, some varieties of tempeh, wheat germ, Accent, Postum, and some forms of yeast. Corn and its other names are discussed in chapter 2.

Following are two lists of flours, gluten and nongluten. Almost all of our recipes require some gluten flour in order to obtain a well-baked and tasty dessert. Generally, you will get a better product using mostly gluten flours. If you are dealing with a gluten allergy then you will have to experiment with nongluten flours and our charts will be of assistance.

GLUTEN FLOURS

Amaranth

Made from the ground grains of the amaranth plant, it is in the Amaranth family (some Amaranth species do not produce edible seeds or grain). It ranges from an off-white to near-black color and has a bland flavor. It works well used as a coating and for baking, and the cooked whole grains may be used in salads. Other varieties of this family are grown for the green leaves, which may be cooked and eaten like spinach and are commonly known as pigweed. The flour is high in protein, calcium, fiber, and B vitamins.

Barley

Made from the ground grain of barley plants, it is in the Grass family. It is commonly used in the manufacture of malt. It has a white color and a mild flavor. It does not work well used as a coating or for thickening. It works well for baking, especially when mixed with a flour that bakes a heavier or denser product, such as rye or buckwheat.

Buckwheat (dark)

Made from the ground grain of the buckwheat plant. In spite of its name, it is not related to the Grass family, but belongs to the Buckwheat family, which includes rhubarb and sorrel. It has a medium brown color and a strong flavor. It works well for a dark crispy coating, and when mixed with other flours will give a solid texture to baked goods. It is not good for thickening or making a roux.

Buckwheat (light)

Made from the unroasted ground grain of the buckwheat plant. It belongs to the same family as the dark buckwheat, and differs only in the preparation of the flour. The flavor can vary from mild to strong, and it has a light brown color. It is good for baking and for use as a coating, producing a medium-weight, dry product, but is not good for thickening or making a roux.

Chickpea or Garbanzo Bean

Made from the dried, ground seeds of the chickpea plant, it is in the Bean family. It has a pale yellow color and a mild flavor. It is only fair for coating, but is excellent for thickening. It can be used for baked goods, but only when it is one-quarter or less of the total flour used (e.g., ¼ cup chickpea flour with ¾ cup other flours).

Kamut

Made from the ground grain of the kamut plant, it is in the Grass family. *Kamut* is the Egyptian word for wheat; it is an ancient, nonhybridized form of wheat. It has an off-white color and a mild flavor. It is good when used for coating, but not for thickening. It works very well for baking.

Millet

Made from the ground grain of the pearl millet plant, it is in the Grass family. It has an off-white color and a very mild flavor. It works for coating, although not as well as some other flours, and does not work well for thickening. It is very good for baking, especially when mixed with other, more glutinous flours (see chart, this chapter).

Oat

Made from the ground kernels of the oat plant, it is in the Grass family. It has an off-white to gray color and a mild flavor. It is very good for coating and thickening. It is also excellent for baking, especially when mixed at a 3:1 ratio with another flour such as arrowroot or potato (e.g., ¾ cup oat flour with ¼ cup potato flour). Note that rolled oats (heated and flattened kernels) are gluten-free.

Potato

Made from the cooked, dried, and ground tuber, it is in the Potato family. It has a white color and no flavor. Potato flour is not recommended for coating, but is very good for thickening. In baking, it works best when mixed with another flour, and can be used for up to half of the total flour used. Note that potato flour and potato starch are different and react in different ways when used. Do not substitute one for the other.

Quinoa

Made from the roasted, ground grain of the quinoa plant, it is in the Goosefoot family. It has an ivory color and a bland flavor. It does not work well for coating or thickening. It works extremely well for baking, especially when mixed with another gluten flour.

Rye

Made from the roasted, ground grain of the rye plant, it is in the Grass family. It has a very dark brown color and a strong, almost yeasty flavor. It works as a coating, but has too strong a flavor to use as a thickener or for making a roux. It works extremely well for breads and some cakes, such as carrot or zucchini, but not as well for cookies or more delicate goods.

Spelt

Made from the ground grain of the spelt plant, it is in the nonhybridized Grass family. It has an ivory to white color and a bland taste. It works extremely well for baking, but not as well for thickening or coating.

Teff

Made from the ground grain of the teff plant, it is in the Grass family. It has a medium to dark color, a coarse texture, and a mild flavor. It works well for baking, but not as well for coating or thickening.

NONGLUTEN FLOURS

Arrowroot

Made from the dried, ground West Indian arrowroot tuber, it is in the Marantaceae family. It has a snow-white color and no flavor. It can be used for a crispy, quick-cooking coating and works very well as a thickening agent. Small amounts may also be added to gluten flours for baking. In catalogs or on packaging, it may be called "flour," "powder," or "starch"; we have found no discernible differences, and in this book we call it arrowroot flour.

Rice

Made from the dried, ground kernels of rice plants, it is in the Grass family. Flours milled from brown and from refined white rice are available; the colors range from white to light brown, and all have a mild flavor. It is not good for coating, unless you are preparing tempura batter. It works best in baked goods when mixed with other flours, and will impart a light, silky texture to the product.

Soy

Made from the roasted, dried, ground soybean, it is in the Bean family. It works well when used for coating, but not for thickening. It is good for baking used at a 1:3 ratio (e.g., ¼ cup soy flour with ¾ cup other flours). Make sure the flour you purchase has been made from already-roasted soybeans. Because soy has a higher oil content than other flours, you may wish to reduce the butter, margarine, or oil called for in a recipe by 1 teaspoon for each ¼ cup soy flour used. It will give a silky, almost puddinglike texture to your baked goods. Soy has also been determined to be a common allergen, so daily use is not recommended.

Based on our experience and from information gleaned from many sources, we have developed the following list.

Most Glutinous Flours	Medium Glutinous Flours	Least Glutinous Flours	Nonglutinous Flours
buckwheat	amaranth	barley	arrowroot
oat	kamut	garbanzo	rice
rye	potato	millet	soy
	quinoa		
	spelt		
	teff		

GENERAL SUBSTITUTIONS AND AMOUNTS IN RECIPES

General Flour Substitution Chart for Any Recipe

For each 1 cup of bleached, enriched flour made from wheat called for in a recipe you may generally substitute one of the following:

¼ cup amaranth flour and ¾ cup oat flour

1 cup–1¼ cups rye flour

¼–½ cup buckwheat flour

⅝–1 cup potato flour

1 cup oat flour

½–⅔ cup barley flour

½ cup potato flour and ½ cup rye flour

⅝ cup rice flour and ⅓ cup rye flour

 cup soy flour plus ¾ cup potato starch

The following chart describes general rules for substituting alternative flours for 1 cup of white or whole-wheat flour.

General Flour Substitution Chart for Baked Goods

Denser Baked Goods (such as loaf cakes, pancakes, and muffins)

1–1¼ cup rye flour

¼–½ cup buckwheat flour

⅝–1 cup potato flour

½ cup potato flour and ½ cup rye flour

⅝ cup rice flour and ⅓ cup rye flour

1 cup soy flour and ¾ cup potato starch

Lighter Baked Goods (such as white or yellow cakes, cupcakes, bar cookies, drop cookies, and piecrusts)

¼ cup amaranth flour and ¾ cup oat flour

½ cup oat flour and ½ cup millet flour

½ cup oat flour and ½ cup spelt flour

½ cup spelt flour and ½ cup amaranth flour

¼ cup soy flour and ¾ cup oat flour

These proportions may not look as if they would work but, due to the different families, classes, and characteristics of these grains, they do work. Please note that all the alternative flours react differently with each other; you may want to experiment to find the best combinations for your own cooking and baking needs. We have included separate charts for each of the recipe chapters that specify the substitutions and combinations of alternative flours that we have discovered work best for cookies, cakes, fruit desserts, and crusts.

One helpful hint is to add a little more leavening, such as baking powder, baking soda, egg or egg substitute, or yeast, if a coarser flour rather than a finer flour is used. A good rule of thumb is 2½ teaspoons of additional baking powder or an equivalent substitute for each 1 cup of coarse flour used.

Another suggestion is to let the batter or dough sit for a few minutes after all the ingredients have been thoroughly mixed to allow the alternative flours to absorb any liquids; this helps the flours expand and rise a little better when baking. As you become more proficient in mixing your favorite recipes and using your favorite flours, you will develop a feel for when your dough is the right consistency for a well-baked product.

Appendix I lists the scientific and family names for the grains and flours referred to in this cookbook. A food family name is a botanical classification of foods that are related first by the flower structure and second by the genetic structure. A person with an allergy to one member of a specific food family may also be allergic to other foods in the same family. If your child is allergic to one food in a particular family, check with your doctor before using other members of that food family.

2 Taking Stock of Other Ingredients

Many of the products commonly used for baking and cooking regularly contain ingredients that may be allergens for your child. This chapter discusses the components of commonly available products and suggests substitutions and alternatives that work just as well. We have found that it is best to buy products from health food stores and manufacturers who can guarantee the purity of their ingredients. But if you do not have easy access to a health food store and need substitutions quickly, we hope this chapter will make your life easier. Check chapter 12 for a list of suppliers who will send products to your home.

COMMON INGREDIENTS AND THEIR SUBSTITUTES

Baking powder

Used as a leavening agent to help baked goods rise. Most baking powders have added cornstarch to keep the powder dry and free-pouring. Many have added albumin (egg whites) to assist the rising process.

Substitute any one of the following for each 1 teaspoon baking powder used in a recipe:

½ teaspoon cream of tartar and ½ teaspoon baking soda

1 teaspoon Featherweight baking powder or any brand that is cereal-free (has no cornstarch)

1 teaspoon cream of tartar, 1 teaspoon bicarbonate of soda, and ½ teaspoon salt (if you are following a recipe that is not in this book, combine for each 1 cup flour used in the recipe)

Baking soda

Sometimes used as a leavening agent to help baked goods rise, but not as commonly used as baking powder. Baking soda has no added ingredients and may be used as is. There are no substitutes necessary.

Butter

Normally used to provide fats to assist baked goods in rising and to add flavor. All cow's-milk butters and most margarines are based on cow's-milk products. Use any one of the following substitutes in equivalent proportions to amounts used in recipes:

> goat's-milk butter (see note under "cow's milk" [page 13] for important details)
>
> soft regular (not firm or low-fat) tofu blended in blender or food processor
>
> nondairy (uses no whey or lactose) noncorn oil margarine
>
> flaxseed, canola, or other acceptable mild-flavored oil
>
> lard
>
> shortening (nondairy, noncorn)

Chocolate

While chocolate candy may have hidden additives, pure baking chocolate and pure cocoa may not be allergic substances for your child. Milk chocolate bars such as Hershey's do not have the egg-white gloss that is normally added to boxed candy for consumer eye appeal. Note, however, that white chocolate is also derived from the cacao bean. If your child has a chocolate allergy, you should check with your doctor before using white chocolate or any cacao-bean derivative. Also, most milk chocolates and some carob products use a dairy derivative and may also use a corn syrup sweetener. You should check their ingredients list carefully. Any product with the word "pareve" or "parave" is guaranteed dairy-free.

Substitute carob powder or carob chips for baking chocolate, cocoa, or chocolate chips in equivalent proportions to amounts used in recipes. Carob is made from the roasted, ground, sticky pulp found in the seed pods of the carob tree; it is in the Bean family. It has a taste very similar to chocolate.

Confectioners' sugar

Finely ground cane sugar. It comes from the Grass family. Normally used to provide a silky, smooth frosting or a less dense baked good. Commercial confectioners' sugars have added cornstarch to ensure a dry and free-flowing product. This is also sometimes called powdered sugar.

To make your own confectioners' sugar: Slowly pour granulated sugar ¼ cup at a time into the top opening of blender or food processor already going on high speed. Empty blender or food processor after each ¼ cup is ground. One-half cup granulated sugar will yield a heaping ½ cup confectioners' sugar. Use the amount called for in the recipe.

Corn

It is in the Grass family. Some other names for corn products used in processed foods include: bran, caramel, cerelose, dextrose, fructose, germ meal, glucose, gluten meal, grits, hominy, HVP (hydrolyzed vegetable protein), Karo, maize, maltodextrin, masa harina, modified food starch, polenta, pozole, sucrose, and xanthan gum.

Cornstarch

A derivative of corn normally used as a thickener for fruit pies, custards, puddings, gravies, stews, and some cakes. For persons with a corn allergy, you may substitute one of the following:

Arrowroot powder, flour, or starch. From a dried ground tuber grown in the West Indies, Florida, or Fiji. Dissolve in a small amount of cold water before using. Use $2/3$ tablespoon arrowroot for each 1 tablespoon cornstarch used in recipe.

Kudzu or kudu powder. From the root of the kudzu vine, it is from the Bean family. The root is pounded and mixed with water. The water is then drained from the starchy silt and the process repeated. Sift out lumps, then dissolve the sifted powder in a small amount of cold water before using. Use $1/3$ to ½ tablespoon kudzu for each 1 tablespoon cornstarch used in recipe.

Potato flour. From cooked, dried, and ground white potatoes. Potatoes are from the Potato family. Use 1 tablespoon potato flour for each 1 tablespoon cornstarch used in recipe.

Potato starch. From raw white potatoes. Potatoes are ground and mixed with water. The starchy silt is then removed and dried. Dissolve in a small amount of cold water before using. Use 1 tablespoon potato starch for each 1 tablespoon cornstarch used in recipe.

Rice flour. Made from cooked, dried, and ground rice kernels (Grass family). Dissolve in a small amount of cold water before using. If possible, purchase "Mochika" or "sweet" rice flour, which is made from a waxier type of rice and thickens better with fewer lumps. Use 1 tablespoon rice flour for each 1 tablespoon cornstarch used in recipe.

Tapioca. From the cooked, ground cassava root. It is from the Spurge family. Depending on the recipe, it may be helpful to dissolve the tapioca pearls in hot or cold water before using; see the container for helpful hints. There are a variety of tapiocas available; small pearled quick-cooking tapioca was used in creating these recipes. Use 4 teaspoons tapioca for each 1 tablespoon cornstarch used in recipe.

Corn syrup

Normally used as a sweetener for caramel desserts, as a clear sweetener and thickener for pies, or the basis for glazes on tarts. Also known by trade and other names as caramel, cerelose, dextrose, fructose, glucose, Karo syrup, maltodextrin, and sucrose.

Substitute 1 cup granulated sugar melted over low heat with ¼ cup water for each 1 cup of corn syrup called for in your recipe.

Cow's milk

Normally used to provide fats to assist baked goods in rising and to provide necessary liquids in batters. Commonly used names for cow's-milk products and derivatives are casein, curd, lactalbumin, lactoglobulin, lactose, sodium caseinate, whey, and rennet. Note that calcium carbonate and calcium lactate are not dairy-derived ingredients. Also, any product with the word "pareve" or "parave" is guaranteed dairy-free.

Substitute any one of the following in equivalent proportions to amounts used in recipes:

almond milk

fruit juices, fruit concentrates, or fruit purees (you may want to slightly increase the fat content in the recipe, using margarine or oil, if you find the baked good does not rise well using a nonfat product) goat's milk*

powdered or dried-milk alternatives such as soy-milk powder, Better Than Milk tofu powder, or Meyenberg goat's-milk powder, reconstituted with water

rice milk

soy milk

Egg and egg whites

Used to thicken puddings and custards; to help baked goods rise; to clear soups, like consommés and bouillons; to make meringues, frostings, marshmallows, and marshmallow sauce; to make mayonnaise, hollandaise, and many salad dressings. Also called *albumin*.

Substitute one of the following for 1 egg:

1 teaspoon Ener-G Egg Replacer (contains white potato starch) dissolved in 2 tablespoons cold water

½ teaspoon baking powder

¼ teaspoon baking powder dissolved in 1 tablespoon cold water

1 tablespoon vinegar

2 egg yolks, carefully separated from the whites

Margarine

Normally used to provide fats to assist baked goods in rising. Many margarines use whey or lactose, both of which are cow's-milk products. Use a nondairy (and noncorn oil, if corn is an allergen) margarine or an acceptable (noncorn) mild-tasting oil. Any product with the word "pareve" or "parave" is guaranteed dairy-free.

---

*Note: Goat's-milk products can sometimes be good substitutes for a person who is sensitive to cow's milk. However, various constituents of cow's milk may also be present in goat's milk because of the similar protein compositions. Determine what is causing the allergic reaction before switching to goat's-milk products. Most of the information readily available about cow's milk concerns milk fat, lactose, casein, and whey. Neither milk fat nor lactose has been shown to cause allergic reactions. A person with an allergy to cow's milk is reacting to either the casein or the whey or both. The casein in cow's milk is similar to the casein in goat's milk. If the reaction can be narrowed down to the casein component, then goat's milk should not be used. The most allergic component in cow's milk is the Beta-lactoglobulin, which is the major milk protein found in whey. The whey in goat's milk seems to be different from the whey in cow's milk. If goat's milk can be tolerated and cow's milk causes a reaction, then the sensitivity is probably to the whey, and the casein can be tolerated. Casein is also found in most soy and almond cheeses. Casein allows the cheese to melt and to

Oil

Normally used to provide fats to assist baked goods in rising and to provide necessary liquids in batters. Many vegetable oils may also contain some corn and/or peanut oil; use a pure type, such as flax or canola oil to be sure you are avoiding allergens. Use an equivalent amount of pure oil as called for in the recipe. A mild-tasting oil will work best as a substitute for butter or margarine in the recipes.

Salt

Normally used as a seasoning in cooked foods and to assist the chemical reaction for helping baked goods rise. Most commercial iodized table salts contain dextrose (a corn product) as a stabilizing ingredient, and many of those also have sodium silicoaluminate, an aluminum by-product, which may concern you as it does us. However, many local grocery stores also carry sea salt and "pickling" or "preserving" salts, which work just as well as table salt for cooking or baking and are dextrose-free and sodium silicoaluminate-free. Some manufacturers offer iodine-free table and cooking salts that do not contain dextrose. Note, however, that kosher or "sour" salt is *not* an acceptable substitute for baking desserts or to replace table salt.

Sweeteners

Used to sweeten and add flavor to foods and baked goods. Many kinds of sweeteners are available in addition to granulated cane sugar. Fruit sweeteners come in many forms, including granulated, powdered, dried, pureed, juiced, juice concentrates, liquid, sauce, and mashed. Having a variety of sweeteners in your pantry to choose from will add interest and flavor variations to your foods. However, depending on the form of sweetener used, the other liquids in your recipe may have to be reduced and/or the dry ingredients increased. We have not tried all of

---

resemble cow's-milk cheese. If casein can be tolerated, then most alternative cheeses are allowable. If casein is the allergen, avoid soy, almond, and other cheeses that contain it. Can a person with cow's-milk allergy tolerate the special milks formulated with the lactose-digesting enzyme? Probably not. Lactose intolerance is often mistakenly confused with a milk allergy. These are two different things. In an allergic reaction, the symptoms are produced when an allergen causes histamines to be released in the body's cells. This release brings on the allergic symptoms. In contrast, lactose intolerance is due to a lack of the lactose-digesting enzyme in the body. Symptoms of lactose intolerance can include stomachache, gas, bloating, and diarrhea. Therefore, the person with a cow's-milk allergy will not be able to tolerate the special milks formulated with the lactose-digesting enzyme.

these sweeteners in our recipes. For equivalent substitutions follow package directions or experiment. See chapter 12 for mail-order sources for most of these items when they are not readily available at your local grocery or health food store.

Aquamill. Made from the naturally sweet sap of the century or maguey plant of the Amaryllis family.

Barley malt. A thick syrup or powder made from barley grains. It has a flavor and consistency similar to molasses. It is in the Grass family.

Beet sugar. Made from the refined and dried syrup of the sugar beet. It is in the Goosefoot family. It can be used in equivalent amounts to replace granulated cane sugar in the recipe.

Brown sugar (light or dark). Made from granulated cane sugar or beet sugar with molasses (from the sugar cane plant). Adds flavor and color. Use it in equivalent amounts to replace granulated sugar in a recipe.

Cane sugar. Made from liquid squeezed from the sugarcane stalks of the Grass family. It is then dried and refined to make granulated sugar. It is the most common sweetener used in baked goods.

Corn sweetener (light or dark). Made from liquid squeezed from corn kernels. Commonly known as corn syrup, cerelose, dextrose, glucose, and Karo syrup, it is in the grass family. It is a very inexpensive sweetener and is used extensively in commercial products such as sodas, breakfast cereals, cookies, and many other items. If this is an allergen, great care must be taken to avoid corn under its many names. If your recipe calls for corn syrup, for each 1 cup used you may substitute 1 cup granulated sugar melted over low heat with ¼ cup water.

Dates and date sugar. Sweeteners made from the fruit of the date tree. It is from the Palm family. Dates must be chopped and blended or food processed before using. Dates and date sugar can be used to replace sugar in equivalent amounts, and both act more like granulated sugar when used in baked goods than other fruit sweeteners or juices do. Use ²/₃ cup blended dates or date sugar for each 1 cup of granulated cane sugar used in recipe.

Fructose. A sugar found in nearly all fruits and honey. It is twice as sweet as granulated cane sugar and is available as a liquid, powder, or tablet. See package directions for substitution information.

Fruit juices and concentrates. Must be thawed before using if frozen. Use full strength (not diluted with water) to replace the liquid in the recipe. This adds both sweetness to the baked good and also the needed acidity for the leavening process.

Fruit purees and whips. Can be purchased or made at home using a blender or food processor. Simply peel and pit larger fruits, or pit berries, and blend or process until smooth. For some berries, such as raspberries, put through a sieve or fine strainer before using. Commonly used fruits include apple, apricot, banana, date, fig, pear, plum, and prune. Fruit purees and whips can greatly improve the texture of many baked goods by helping to bind crumbly desserts.

Granulated sugar. See cane or beet sugar, above.

Honey. Two and one-half times sweeter than granulated cane sugar. Raw, unfiltered, locally produced honey is usually best for people with allergies. Decrease the liquid called for in the recipe by ¼ cup for each 1 cup of honey. For example, if the recipe calls for 1 cup milk and 2 cups of sugar, use ¾ cup milk and ¾–1 cup honey, to taste.

Maple sugar and syrup. Comes from the sap of trees in the Maple family. It is a fine replacement for granulated cane sugar. Since many types of commercial maple syrup and "breakfast" syrups and some maple sugars contain corn sweeteners, be sure you are buying a pure maple syrup or sugar. Decrease the liquid called for by ¼ cup for each 1 cup of maple syrup. For example, if the recipe uses 1 cup milk and 1 cup sugar, use ¾ cup milk and 1 cup maple syrup. Use an equivalent amount of maple sugar for the amount of granulated sugar used in the recipe.

Molasses. The syrupy residue left from the process that produces granulated sugar from sugar canes. It has a strong, sweet, but almost sulfuric taste that comes through clearly in baked goods. It is not recommended as the only substitute for cane sugar or other sweeteners when cooking or baking, but is tasty in many foods when used in conjunction with other sweeteners.

Rice sugar, rice syrup, and rice powder. Produced from processed rice grains. Rice is from the Grass family. It has a light, smooth texture and a very mild flavor. Use an equivalent amount of rice sugar for the amount of granulated cane sugar in your recipe.

Stevia. A sweet herb, *Stevia rebaudiana*, found in Ecuador. It is available as a brownish or a white powder or as a liquid. It is a very concentrated sweetener and you may want to dissolve it in the recipe's liquid for better distribution. Use approximately ¹/₃ cup Stevia for each 1 cup granulated cane sugar.

Turbinado. A by-product of the granulated sugarcane process. It is a less refined sugarcane sweetener, usually coarse in texture and with a molasseslike flavor. It may be used in equivalent amounts to replace granulated sugar.

Vanilla

Normally used to provide flavoring for baked goods. From the vainilla ("little scabbard" in Spanish) orchid in the Orchid family. Most commercial vanilla extracts and vanilla flavorings have corn syrup added as a sweetener. Most also use grain (corn or wheat) alcohol as the base in the extraction process.

Substitute any of the following in equivalent amounts used in a recipe:

   acquavit (made from rice, yeast)

   arak (made from oats, coconut, cane, yeast)

   brandy (made from grapes)

   okolehao (made from rice, taro, cane)

   rum, U. S. or Jamaican (made from grapes, cane, yeast)

   saki (made from rice and yeast)

   scotch, unblended single malt (does not contain corn, wheat, or potato)

   vodka (made from potatoes)

   very strong cold coffee

To make your own vanilla extract: Chop 1 pound vanilla beans and place them in a large container; add ½ gallon of any acceptable clear alcohol; let steep for at least four weeks. Strain out the chopped beans and store the vanilla extract in a tightly sealed jar. Or slice 2 vanilla beans lengthwise, scrape out the tiny seeds and add them to your mixture before cooking or baking. Or slice 1 vanilla bean lengthwise and add it to the sauce or custard as it is cooking; remember to remove before serving. You can make vanilla sugar and use in equivalent amounts in recipes by placing 1 whole vanilla bean in a large covered jar with granulated sugar, tightly sealed. The vanilla flavor will intensify the longer you leave the bean in the sugar.

Vinegar

Normally used with other ingredients to assist baked goods in rising. White vinegars are distilled from a variety of grains, fruits, and vegetables, while cider (brown) vinegar normally uses apple cider as its base. Since cider vinegar usually has as high a level of acidity (the important factor in baking, cooking, and pickling) as white vinegar, people with grain and potato allergies may use cider vinegar with confidence.

BAKING INGREDIENTS SUBSTITUTION CHARTS

The following chart gives alternatives for common allergens in baking ingredients. See pages 9–18 for a more detailed description of each ingredient. Use the equivalent amount of the substitute ingredient unless otherwise specified.

Please be sure that the substitutes you choose do not contain the allergens you are trying to avoid. This is particularly important with multiple allergies. For example, when avoiding cow's milk and corn, be sure the carob chips you are using do not contain whey or corn syrup sweeteners.

Alternative Ingredients Chart

Common Ingredient	Allergen-Free Substitution
1 teaspoon baking powder	½ teaspoon cream of tartar and ½ teaspoon baking soda 1 teaspoon Featherweight baking powder
butter	goat's-milk butter nondairy (whey- and lactose-free), noncorn oil margarine mild-tasting corn-free oil soft tofu (not low-fat), mashed or blended
chocolate	carob
confectioners' sugar	homemade (see recipe, page 11)

Common Ingredient	Allergen-Free Substitution
1 tablespoon cornstarch	$2/3$ tablespoon arrowroot flour
	$1/3$–$1/2$ tablespoon kudzu powder
	1 tablespoon potato flour or potato starch
	1 tablespoon rice flour
	4 teaspoons tapioca
1 cup corn syrup	1 cup granulated sugar melted with $1/4$ cup water
cow's milk	almond milk
	fruit juices, concentrates, or purees
	goat's milk
	reconstituted nondairy powdered milk
	rice milk
	soy milk
1 egg	1 teaspoon Ener-G Egg Replacer mixed with 2 tablespoons cold water
	$1/2$ teaspoon baking powder
	$1/4$ teaspoon baking powder mixed with 1 tablespoon cold water
	1 tablespoon vinegar
	2 egg yolks, carefully separated from the whites
margarine	nondairy (whey- and lactose-free), noncorn oil margarine
	mild-tasting corn-free oil
salt	sea salt
vanilla	acquavit
	arak
	brandy
	coffee, very strong cold
	homemade (see recipe, page 17)
	okolehao
	rum, U. S. or Jamaican
	sake
	scotch, unblended single malt
	vodka

The following chart lists common ingredients and their corresponding allergens. Refer to pages 9–18 for a detailed description of each ingredient and why it may be an allergen for your child.

Items and Allergens Chart

Item	Allergen					
	Wheat	Egg	Corn	Dairy	Nut	Chocolate
flour	X		X			
baking powder			X			
butter				X		
chocolate		X	X	X		X
confectioners' sugar			X			
cornstarch			X			
corn syrup			X			
cow's milk				X		
egg		X				
margarine			X	X		
oil			X		X	
salt			X			
vanilla	X		X			
vinegar			X			
yeast	X					

The following items are necessary in the allergen-free kitchen. Most of these items are readily available at supermarkets or health food stores. If you have difficulty finding any of these products at your local store, check chapter 12 for a listing of manufacturers and suppliers to buy from directly.

Stocking Your Pantry

baking powder	margarine
baking soda	oil
chocolate or carob chips	potato starch
cocoa or carob powder	sea salt
cow's-milk alternatives	tapioca, pearled
Ener-G Egg Replacer	vanilla extract
flour alternatives	vinegar, cider

The following list comprises most of the basic equipment needed, but not required, for the recipes in this book.

The Well-Equipped Kitchen

blender

bowls, assorted sizes for mixing batters and doughs, plastic and glass

bundt pan (optional)

cake pans, 8-inch round or square and 9" x 13" rectangular

casserole dishes, 1½-quart and 2½-quart, microwave-safe in any shape, with covers

cookie sheets, preferably insulated sheets

cupcake papers

cupcake tins, one large 6-well tin and one regular 12-well tin

electric mixer (optional)

food processor (optional)

grater

jars with lids, 8-ounce and 16-ounce

jars for canning with new lids and rings, 8-ounce

knife, blunt table

knife, sharp

ladle, large

loaf pan, 5" x 9"

measuring cups, from ¼ cup to 1 cup

measuring spoons, from ⅛ teaspoon to 1 tablespoon

microwave oven

microwave-safe dish, 8-inch square

pastry cutter (optional)

peeler or paring knife

pie pan, 9-inch

pot, 2-gallon or larger

saucepans, small, medium, and large, non-aluminum with covers

sifter

skillet

spatulas, metal and rubber

springform pan, 9-inch

rolling pin

spoons, large slotted and large mixing

strainer

tart pan, 11-inch (optional)

toothpicks (the longer and larger sandwich toothpicks are easier to use when checking for doneness)

waffle iron (optional)

3 Cakes and Frostings Without Fear

*H*aving now lived through five years' worth of birthdays, countless parties, and school celebrations, we finally admit that cakes and cupcakes are a fact of life.

Adapting our existing ingredients and our "stop at the bakery on the way home from work" lifestyle was a *major* change. We changed from whole-wheat and white flours to amaranth, barley, buckwheat, kamut, oat, potato, quinoa, rice, rye, soy, and spelt flours; we retraced our baking roots from cake mixes back to scratch; we tasted our way from 2 percent and skim milk to soy, rice, almond, and goat's milks; we mixed, kneaded, beat, and burned our way from simple recipes to line-by-line substitutions until we had desserts that were not just edible and pretty, but delicious, too!

Light, airy cakes result from gases produced by leavening agents trapped inside flours, from air beaten into an egg or into a butter-and-sugar mixture, or from a combination of the two. Because our flours have different textures and gluten contents than the usual bleached, enriched flour made from wheat, and because we do not use whole eggs, we must make a special effort to create these trapped pockets of gases. The recipes call for mixing ingredients and beating batters by hand with a large spoon, preferably wooden; you may choose to use an electric mixer set on the lower settings. We have found, however, that using a food processor or a blender will make a batter that is too sticky and gluey and does not bake well. You may want to take a little extra time to cream the butter, margarine, or oil with the sweetener very thoroughly, as this will create a lot of little air pockets. You will also want to remember to have egg yolks and all liquids at room temperature. Adding cold ingredients forces out the air and allows the butter, margarine, or oil to harden. Sifting the Ener-G Egg Replacer powder, baking soda, or baking powder with the flours before adding them to the creamed mixture will ensure an even distribution of leavening agents and create uniform air pockets as the cake bakes, instead of producing only several large holes. Finally, while our recipes call for mixing flours into the batter completely, too much mixing will beat the air pockets out of the creamed ingredients.

We found that pan sizes were variable: if the recipe calls for a 9" x 13" pan, but you only have two 8-inch pans, go ahead! You might find you like the cake better as a layer cake. All of the cake recipes call for an 8-inch cake pan that can be either square or round, or you can use a 9-inch pan and the cooking time is the same. We also found that, unlike many commercial mixes and recipes, almost all of our cake recipes easily convert to cupcakes. When noted in the recipe that the cake can also be a cupcake dessert, use one 12-cup tin, lined with cupcake papers, and fill each paper one-half to two-thirds full with the batter. Just be sure to watch the clock, peek into your oven several times, and start the toothpick test earlier than required for cakes, as cupcakes bake more quickly.

We also found that mixing a gluten flour, such as oat or barley with a "finer" nongluten flour such as rice or soy makes a lighter, silkier cake. Many of our recipes list a variety of ingredients for you to choose from; the ingredient listed first in each line is the one with which we had the best success, but the alternatives will also work. If there is only one ingredient listed on a particular line, we have not found (or do not need) an acceptable alternative for it. Please feel free to try your own combinations, and remember that as you get used to the different ways the substitute flours interact, you will become a pro at achieving your desired results.

Each recipe suggests a specific baking time. However, due to different altitudes and a range of oven temperature calibrations, we recommend you use a toothpick to determine when a cake is done. A cake is fully baked when a toothpick inserted into the center of the cake comes out clean. Dough clinging to the toothpick means the batter is not quite baked. Wait until the recommended baking time has elapsed, and begin checking at one-minute intervals if your first toothpick is doughy. Cakes will also start to pull away from the sides of the baking pan when almost baked. This is a good "eyeball" measure of doneness.

When fruits or berries are called for, you may use fresh or frozen. Frozen berries and small pieces of fruits will thaw and cook in the batter. Also, please note that whenever spices are an ingredient, we are using dried, ground spices—not whole. If whole or fresh spices are required, they will be specifically noted as such in that recipe.

Finally, since alternative-flour cakes are more fragile than bleached, enriched wheat-flour cakes, try to serve them from the baking pan whenever possible to lessen the chance of the cake breaking or crumbling. You might want to try using parchment paper, cornfree waxed paper, or oiled brown paper to line the bottom of your cake pans before baking, as this will help the cake turn out more easily.

Cake Flour Chart

These are suggested combinations of flours that work well for light-tasting and less dense cakes. All combinations are for 1 cup.
NO means the flour alone or that combination of flours is not appropriate for a good cake.
OK means the flour may be used by itself and does not require another flour in addition to it.
ANY COMB. means any ratio of the two flours that adds up to 1 cup will make a good cake.

	Amaranth	Barley	Chickpea/Garbanzo	Millet	Oat
Amaranth	OK	up to ¼ cup barley with ¾ cup or more amaranth	up to ¼ cup chickpea with ¾ cup or more amaranth	up to ¼ cup millet with ¾ cup or more amaranth	ANY COMB.
Barley	up to ¼ cup barley with ¾ cup or more amaranth	NO	NO	up to ¼ cup barley and up to ½ cup millet with ½ cup or more oat or spelt	up to ½ cup barley with ½ cup or more oat
Chickpea/ Garbanzo	up to ¼ cup chickpea with ¾ cup or more amaranth	NO	NO	up to ¼ cup chickpea and up to ¼ cup millet with ½ cup or more oat or spelt	up to ½ cup chickpea with ½ cup or more oat or spelt

	Amaranth	Barley	Chickpea/Garbanzo	Millet	Oat
Millet	up to ¼ cup millet with ¾ cup or more amaranth	up to ¼ cup millet and up to ¼ cup barley with ½ cup or more oat or spelt	up to ¼ cup millet and up to ¼ cup chickpea with ½ cup or more oat or spelt	NO	up to ½ cup millet with ½ cup or more oat
Oat	ANY COMB.	up to ½ cup barley with ½ cup or more oat	up to ½ cup chickpea with ½ cup or more oat	up to ½ cup millet with ½ cup or more oat	OK
Potato	up to ¼ cup potato with ¾ cup or more amaranth	up to ¼ cup potato and up to ¼ cup barley with ½ cup or more oat or spelt	NO	up to ¼ cup potato and up to ¼ cup millet with ½ cup or more oat or spelt	up to ¼ cup potato with ¾ cup or more oat
Quinoa	ANY COMB.	up to ⅓ cup barley with ⅔ cup or more quinoa	up to ⅓ cup chickpea with ⅔ cup or more quinoa	up to ½ cup millet with ½ cup or more quinoa	ANY COMB.
Rice	up to ¼ cup rice with ¾ cup or more amaranth	up to ¼ cup rice and up to ¼ cup barley with ½ cup or more quinoa, oat or spelt	up to ¼ cup rice and up to ¼ cup chickpea with ½ cup or more quinoa, oat or spelt	up to ¼ cup rice and up to ¼ cup millet with ½ cup or more quinoa, oat or spelt	up to ⅓ cup rice with ⅔ cup or more oat

	Amaranth	Barley	Chickpea/Garbanzo	Millet	Oat
Soy	up to $1/3$ cup soy with $2/3$ cup or more amaranth	up to $1/4$ cup soy and up to $1/4$ cup barley with $1/2$ cup or more quinoa, oat or spelt	up to $1/4$ cup soy and up to $1/4$ cup chickpea with $1/2$ cup or more quinoa, oat or spelt	up to $1/4$ cup soy and up to $1/4$ cup millet with $1/2$ cup or more quinoa, oat or spelt	up to $1/3$ cup soy with $2/3$ cup or more oat
Spelt	ANY COMB.	up to $1/2$ cup barley with $1/2$ cup or more spelt	up to $1/2$ cup chickpea with $1/2$ cup or more spelt	up to $1/2$ cup millet with $1/2$ cup or more spelt	ANY COMB.

	Potato	Quinoa	Rice	Soy	Spelt
Amaranth	up to $1/4$ cup potato with $3/4$ cup or more amaranth	ANY COMB.	up to $1/4$ cup rice with $3/4$ cup or more amaranth	up to $1/3$ cup soy with $2/3$ cup or more amaranth	ANY COMB.
Barley	up to $1/4$ cup potato and up to $1/4$ cup barley with $1/2$ cup or more quinoa, oat or spelt	up to $1/3$ cup barley with $2/3$ cup or more quinoa	up to $1/4$ cup rice and up to $1/4$ cup barley with $1/2$ cup or more quinoa, oat or spelt	up to $1/4$ cup soy and up to $1/4$ cup barley with $1/2$ cup or more quinoa, oat or spelt	up to $1/2$ cup barley with $1/2$ cup or more spelt
Chickpea\ Garbanzo	NO	up to $1/3$ cup chickpea with $2/3$ cup or more quinoa	up to $1/4$ cup rice and up to $1/4$ cup chickpea with $1/2$ cup or more quinoa, oat or spelt	up to $1/4$ cup soy and up to $1/4$ cup chickpea with $1/2$ cup or more quinoa, oat or spelt	up to $1/2$ cup chickpea with $1/2$ cup or more spelt

	Potato	Quinoa	Rice	Soy	Spelt
Millet	up to ¼ cup potato and up to ¼ cup millet with ½ cup or more quinoa, oat or spelt	up to ½ cup millet with ½ cup or more quinoa	up to ¼ cup rice and up to ¼ cup millet with ½ cup or more quinoa, oat or spelt	up to ¼ cup soy and up to ¼ cup millet with ½ cup or more quinoa, oat or spelt	up to ½ cup millet with ½ cup or more spelt
Oat	up to ¼ cup potato with ¾ cup or more oat	ANY COMB.	up to $\frac{1}{3}$ cup rice with $\frac{2}{3}$ cup or more oat	up to $\frac{1}{3}$ cup soy with $\frac{2}{3}$ cup or more oat	ANY COMB.
Potato	NO	up to ¼ cup potato with ¾ cup or more quinoa	up to ¼ cup rice and up to ¼ cup potato with ½ cup or more quinoa, oat or spelt	up to ¼ cup soy and up to ¼ cup potato with ½ cup or more quinoa, oat or spelt	up to ¼ cup potato with ¾ cup or more spelt
Quinoa	up to ¼ cup potato with ¾ cup or more quinoa	OK	up to ¼ cup rice with ¾ cup or more quinoa	up to ¼ cup soy with ¾ cup or more quinoa	ANY COMB.
Rice	up to ¼ cup potato and up to ¼ cup rice with ½ cup or more quinoa, oat or spelt	up to ¼ cup rice with ¾ cup or more quinoa	NO	up to ¼ cup soy and up to ¼ cup rice with ½ cup or more quinoa, oat or spelt	up to ¼ cup rice with ¾ cup or more spelt

	Potato	Quinoa	Rice	Soy	Spelt
Soy	up to ¼ cup potato and up to ¼ cup soy with ½ cup or more quinoa, oat or spelt	up to ¼ cup soy with ¾ cup or more quinoa	up to ¼ cup rice and up to ¼ cup soy with ½ cup or more quinoa, oat or spelt	NO	up to ¼ cup soy with ¾ cup or more spelt
Spelt	up to ¼ cup potato with ¾ cup or more spelt	ANY COMB.	up to ¼ cup rice with ¾ cup or more spelt	up to ¼ cup soy with ¾ cup or more spelt	OK

Banana Loaf Cake

This recipe is excellent for cupcakes, too!

Makes one 5" x 9" loaf cake or 12 cupcakes

¹/₃ cup maple syrup

½ teaspoon vanilla extract

½ cup mashed bananas

½ cup water *or* cow's milk *or* soy milk

2–3 tablespoons butter *or* margarine *or* mild-tasting oil *

2 teaspoons cinnamon

2 teaspoons baking powder

1 cup oat flour

½ cup barley flour *or* potato flour

½ cup rice flour *or* soy flour

*If you are trying to reduce the amount of fat in your diet, you can omit the butter or margarine or oil and still achieve delicious results.

Preheat oven to 325°F. Grease and flour one 5" x 9" loaf pan. For cupcakes, line one 12-cup cupcake tin with cupcake papers.

Combine maple syrup, vanilla, mashed bananas, water or milk, and butter or margarine or oil. Mix well with spoon by hand or with an electric mixer on low. Add cinnamon, and baking powder and mix well. Add oat flour with barley or potato flour. Add rice or soy flour and mix well.

This is a very thick batter. If you feel uncomfortable with the stiffness of the batter, add 1 tablespoon water or milk and mix in well. Spoon into loaf pan.

Bake for 70 minutes or until inserted toothpick comes out clean. If making cupcakes, fill each paper two-thirds full and bake approximately 45 minutes or until inserted toothpick comes out clean.

Serve warm, or cooled and frosted.

Microwave Blueberry Upside-Down Cake

Makes one 8-inch cake

1 tablespoon butter *or* margarine (for the baking dish)

Fruit Topping

2 cups blueberries, rinsed

1 teaspoon arrowroot flour

1 teaspoon grated lemon peel

¼ teaspoon sugar

Cake

½ cup sugar

4 tablespoons softened butter *or* softened margarine

1 teaspoon vanilla extract

½ teaspoon Ener-G Egg Replacer powder

⅓ cup cow's milk *or* soy milk

1 cup oat flour

½ teaspoon baking powder

In a microwave-safe 8-inch baking dish, heat 1 tablespoon butter or margarine for 35 seconds on HIGH.

For the topping: In a large bowl, stir blueberries, arrowroot flour, lemon peel, and sugar until well mixed. Spoon the berry mixture evenly onto the melted butter or margarine in baking dish.

For the cake: Using the same bowl, mix the sugar with the softened butter or margarine until creamy. Add vanilla and Ener-G Egg Replacer powder; mix well. Add milk; beat well. Add oat flour and baking powder; mix well. Spoon the batter evenly over blueberries, using the back of the spoon to pat down and level the dough surface.

Microwave, uncovered, for 8 minutes on MEDIUM, then for 3–5 minutes on HIGH until inserted toothpick comes out clean. Rotate several times during cooking.

Cool for 10 minutes, then lay a large plate over the crust's surface and turn the dish over, tapping several times to loosen berries. Spoon any berries left in cooking dish onto the cake.

Carrot Cake

So you want to serve something delicious, but don't want to give up that nagging urge to be health-conscious? Carrot cake fills your needs, with or without the cream cheese frosting.

Makes one bundt cake or two 8-inch cakes

4 egg yolks

½ cup mild-tasting oil

5 tablespoons hot water

1½ cups grated carrot

1½ teaspoons baking powder

½ teaspoon baking soda

½ teaspoon salt

1 teaspoon each ground nutmeg, cinnamon, and cloves

6 teaspoons Ener-G Egg Replacer powder

1 cup sugar

½ cup oat flour

½ cup barley flour

½ cup soy flour *or* potato flour

Preheat oven to 350°F. Grease and flour one bundt cake pan or two 8-inch cake pans.

Mix egg yolks, oil, and hot water well. Add grated carrots and mix well. Add baking powder, baking soda, salt, nutmeg, cinnamon, cloves, and Ener-G Egg Replacer powder; mix well. Add sugar; mix well. Add oat flour, barley flour, and soy or potato flour; mix well for another 5–10 minutes. Pour into cake pan.

Bake for 60–70 minutes or until inserted toothpick comes out clean.

Cool and frost with cream cheese frosting if desired (see Index).

Chocolate Cake

This is a simple one-bowl cake. It doubles easily for a large 9" x 13" cake.

Makes one 8-inch cake or 12 cupcakes

½ teaspoon baking soda

1 cup cooled black coffee

2 teaspoons vanilla extract

2 teaspoons baking powder

½ teaspoon salt

½ cup sugar

6 heaping tablespoons carob powder *or* cocoa powder

6 tablespoons softened butter *or* softened margarine *or* mild-tasting oil

½ cup oat flour

¾ cup flour (e.g., any one or combination of barley, rice, soy, *or* millet; *or* see chart, this chapter)

Preheat oven to 350°F. Using some extra carob or cocoa powder, flour one ungreased 8-inch cake pan. If making cupcakes, line one 12-cup cupcake tin with cupcake papers.

In a large bowl, mix baking soda and coffee; add vanilla and baking powder and mix well. The batter will foam at this point: do not worry! Add salt, sugar, and carob or cocoa powder; mix well. Add butter or margarine or oil; mix well. Add flours; mix well.

If your batter is really stiff and unworkable, add a little water by teaspoonfuls until you like the consistency, but it should be a fairly thick batter. Spoon into cake pan.

Bake for 35 minutes or until inserted toothpick comes out clean. If you are making cupcakes, start doing a toothpick check at 25 minutes.

To serve, place a paper lace doily on the top of the baked cake, dust with powdered sugar, and remove the doily. Or cool completely and frost.

Chocolate—Sour Cream Cake

This recipe was made as cupcakes for a child's birthday party, and the adults ate them all up! For a special treat, 10 ounces of mini-chocolate chips were added, and it was almost too rich.

Makes two 8-inch cakes or one 9" x 13" cake or 16 cupcakes

⅔ cup softened butter *or* softened margarine *or* mild-tasting oil

2 cups sour cream *or* plain yogurt, dairy or nondairy

1 teaspoon vanilla extract

3 teaspoons Ener-G Egg Replacer powder mixed with 1 tablespoon cold water

1 teaspoon salt

1¾ cups sugar

½ teaspoon baking soda

¾ cup carob powder *or* cocoa powder

1¾ cups flour (e.g., ½ cup barley, ¼ cup rice, and 1 cup oat; *or* see chart, this chapter)

10 ounces mini-chocolate chips *or* mini-carob chips (optional)

Preheat oven to 350°F. Grease and flour two 8-inch cake pans or one 9" x 13" cake pan. If making cupcakes, line cupcake tin with cupcake papers.

In a large bowl, beat butter or margarine or oil, sour cream or yogurt, and vanilla. Add Ener-G Egg Replacer powder, already mixed with cold water; beat in well. Add salt, sugar, and baking soda; mix well. Add carob or cocoa powder; mix well. Add flour; mix well. If you are using mini-chips, mix them in at this point. Pour into cake pan(s).

Bake for 40–45 minutes or until inserted toothpick comes out clean. If you are making cupcakes, start doing a toothpick check at 30 minutes.

Cool, frost if desired, and serve.

Emergency Carob Cake

One day during breakfast, I realized my five-year-old son had no cake to take with him to a birthday party that afternoon. It seemed so unfair for him to go to a party and not have cake to eat. This cake was mixed together and into the oven in 10 minutes. He loved it!

Makes one 9" x 13" cake or 16–18 cupcakes

2 cups sugar *or* 1⅓ cups fructose

3 cups flour (e.g., 1 cup oat, 1 cup barley, and 1 cup potato; *or* see chart, this chapter)

½ cup carob powder *or* cocoa powder

2 teaspoons baking soda

1 teaspoon baking powder

2 tablespoons cider vinegar

⅔ cup mild-tasting oil *or* butter *or* margarine

2 teaspoons vanilla extract

2 cups cold water

Preheat oven to 350°F. Grease and flour one 9" x 13" cake pan. If making cupcakes, line cupcake tin with cupcake papers.

Mix sugar or fructose, flour, carob or cocoa powder, baking soda, baking powder, and vinegar. Add oil or butter or margarine, vanilla, and water, mixing continually until smooth. Pour into cake pan.

Bake for 35–40 minutes or until inserted toothpick comes out clean. If you are making cupcakes, begin toothpick check at 20 minutes.

Mini-Chocolate Chip Cake

Everyone who has tried it has loved this cake!

Makes one 8-inch cake

¼ cup softened butter *or* softened margarine *or* mild-tasting oil

⅓ cup water *or* cow's milk *or* soy milk *or* almond milk

1 teaspoon vanilla extract

1 cup light or dark brown sugar, packed

3 teaspoons baking powder

1 teaspoon Ener-G Egg Replacer powder

1 cup oat flour

½ cup barley flour

½ cup rice flour *or* soy flour

10 ounces mini-chocolate chips *or* mini-carob chips

Preheat oven to 375°F. Grease one 8-inch cake pan.

Combine butter or margarine or oil, water or milk, and vanilla and mix well. Add brown sugar, baking powder, and Ener-G Egg Replacer powder; mix well. Add the flour ½ cup at a time, mixing well after each addition. Add mini-chocolate or carob chips; mix well. Pour into cake pan.

Bake for 30 minutes or until inserted toothpick comes out clean. Cool, frost if desired, and serve.

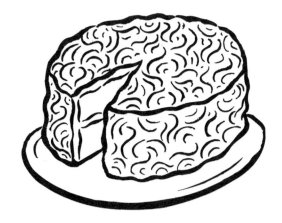

Pineapple Banana Upside-Down Cake

Topping

2 tablespoons margarine *or* butter *or* mild-tasting oil

¼ cup chopped almonds *or* macadamia nuts *or* your choice

$1/3$ cup light or dark brown sugar, packed

Fruit

8 ounces canned chunk or crushed pineapple, drained

1 banana, sliced

Cake

1 cup sugar *or* ¾ cup honey

½ cup softened butter *or* softened margarine *or* mild-tasting oil

1 teaspoon vanilla extract

$2/3$ cup cow's milk *or* soy milk *or* rice milk

2 egg yolks *or* 3 tablespoons Ener-G Egg Replacer powder

½ cup flour (e.g., any one or combination of oat *or* spelt; *or* see chart, this chapter)

¾ cup uncooked oats

1 tablespoon baking powder

Preheat oven to 350°F. Use one 8-inch ungreased cake pan.

Place topping ingredients into the cake pan; place the pan in the heated oven and leave it until the brown sugar has begun to liquify (usually a few minutes). Remove pan from oven. Stir until all three ingredients are well mixed. Arrange the pineapple chunks and banana slices evenly on top of the topping mixture; set pan aside.

In a large bowl, beat sugar or honey, butter or margarine or oil, and vanilla until smooth. Add milk and egg yolks or Ener-G Egg Replacer powder and beat until smooth. Slowly add flour, oats, and baking powder, beating well to keep the batter smooth. Pour slowly and evenly over the fruit mixture in the baking pan.

Bake 45–50 minutes or until inserted toothpick comes out clean. Slide a blunt knife around the inside edges of the baking pan until the cake is loosened from the sides of the pan. Cover the baking pan completely with a large plate and, using oven mitts, hold the plate on tightly and flip the cake upside down onto the plate. Scrape out any remaining topping from the pan and spread it onto the cake top.

Cool before serving.

"Sand" Cake

This favorite and easy recipe is a lifesaver. With only four weeks to create a birthday cake for my son's fifth birthday without using egg or wheat, the "sand" cake was frantically devised from a regular cake recipe that used a little potato flour along with white cake flour; I substituted barley and oat flours for the white flour, along with other allergen-free changes.

Makes one 8-inch cake

½ cup potato flour
½ cup barley flour
1 cup oat flour
1 cup sugar
3 teaspoons baking powder
1 teaspoon Ener-G Egg Replacer powder
²/₃ cup mild-tasting oil *or* shortening *or* softened butter *or* softened margarine
¹/₃ cup water *or* cow's milk *or* soy milk *or* rice milk *or* almond milk
1 teaspoon lemon extract *or* grated lemon peel

Preheat oven to 375°F. Grease one 8-inch cake pan.

Mix potato, barley, and oat flours well. Add sugar, baking powder, and Ener-G Egg Replacer powder; mix well. Cream in oil or shortening or butter or margarine; mix well. Add water or milk and lemon extract or peel; mix well. At this point, the batter should be like smooth mashed potatoes, but not have a really stiff texture. If your batter seems a little too stiff or dry, add more liquid (milk or water) by teaspoonfuls until you are happy with the batter's consistency. Pour into cake pan.

Bake for 30 minutes or until the middle is firm to your touch.

Cool, frost if desired, and serve.

Variation: You can substitute orange extract, grated orange peel, or almond extract for the lemon extract or peel.

Sponge Cake

This is a favorite at family gatherings because it appeals to a wide variety of tastes.

Makes one 8-inch cake

1 cup oat flour

½ cup barley flour *or* potato flour

½ cup millet flour

1 cup sugar

3 teaspoons baking powder

1 teaspoon Ener-G Egg Replacer powder

¼ cup plus 1 tablespoon mild-tasting oil *or* softened butter *or* softened margarine

1 teaspoon grated lemon peel *or* orange peel (optional)

½ cup cold water

Preheat oven to 375°F. Grease one 8-inch cake pan.

Mix oat, barley or potato, and millet flours well. Add sugar, baking powder, and Ener-G Egg Replacer powder; mix well. Cream in oil or butter or margarine and lemon or orange peel; mix well. Add water; mix well until smooth. This is a somewhat stiff batter, more like a dough. If you feel it is too heavy and doughy, add cold water or any other cold liquid by teaspoonfuls until you have a workable batter, but it should still be "doughy" rather than "liquidy." Pat batter into cake pan.

Bake for 35 minutes or until inserted toothpick comes out clean. Cool, and serve.

Holiday Honey Cake

This cake can be made well ahead of time. It keeps for weeks, and it toasts up great!

Makes one 5" x 9" loaf cake

1 cup rye flour

1 cup spelt flour

½ teaspoon baking soda

2 teaspoons baking powder

1 teaspoon cinnamon

$\frac{1}{3}$ cup honey

½ cup sugar

¾ cup water

$\frac{1}{3}$ cup softened butter *or* softened margarine *or* mild-tasting oil

Preheat oven to 350°F. Use one 5" x 9" loaf pan, ungreased and unfloured.

Mix rye and spelt flours with the baking soda, baking powder, and cinnamon; set aside. In a microwave-safe dish or in a small saucepan, mix honey, sugar, and water; heat slowly until small bubbles begin to appear. Remove from the microwave or stovetop; in the dish or saucepan add the butter or margarine or oil; beat until well mixed. Pour this into the flour mixture and beat for 10 minutes. Pour batter into loaf pan.

Bake for 40 minutes or until inserted toothpick comes out clean and the top of the cake has begun to crack.

For the best flavor, cool completely after baking, place in a plastic bag, and refrigerate for three days before serving.

Variation: You may use small amounts of soy, barley, or millet flours in place of some of the rye and spelt flours for a silkier cake. You can also make this a spice cake by reducing the cinnamon to ½ teaspoon and adding $\frac{1}{8}$ teaspoon each of ginger, allspice, and cloves.

Vinegar Cake

*This is an old-fashioned recipe that is really delicious
and doesn't require a bowl.*

Makes one 8-inch cake

1½ cups flour (e.g., 1 cup oat and ½ cup barley, rice, *or* spelt; *or* see chart, this chapter)

1 cup sugar

3 tablespoons cocoa powder *or* carob powder

1 teaspoon baking soda

½ teaspoon salt

5 tablespoons melted butter *or* melted margarine *or* mild-tasting oil

1 tablespoon cider vinegar

1 teaspoon vanilla extract

1 cup cold water

12 ounces carob chips *or* chocolate chips *or* 6 carob candy bars *or* chocolate candy bars (optional)

Preheat oven to 350°F. Use one 8-inch cake pan, ungreased and unfloured.

In the cake pan, mix together the flour, sugar, cocoa or carob powder, baking soda, and salt. Make three well-spaced holes in the dry mixture with your finger; pour butter or margarine or oil into the first hole, pour vinegar into the second hole, and pour vanilla into the third hole. Pour the cold water over all the mixture; then stir with a fork just until smooth.

Bake for 25–35 minutes or until an inserted toothpick comes out clean.

Variation: Immediately after removing the baked cake from the oven, sprinkle carob or chocolate chips evenly over the top of the cake, or cover the top of the baked cake with a single layer of the chocolate or carob bars. Return the cake to the oven (which has now been turned off) for another 2–3 minutes until the chocolate or carob layer is melted. Cool and serve.

Wacky Cake by Grammy

*This recipe can easily be doubled and baked in a 9" x 13"
lightly greased and floured cake pan.*

Makes one 8-inch cake

1½ cups flour (e.g., 1 cup
oat *or* spelt and ½ cup barley *or* millet; *or* see chart,
this chapter)

⅓ cup carob powder *or*
cocoa powder

1 cup sugar

½ teaspoon salt

1 teaspoon baking soda

8 tablespoons melted butter
or melted margarine *or*
mild-tasting oil

2 tablespoons cider vinegar

2 teaspoons vanilla extract

2 cups water

Preheat oven to 350°F. Use one greased and floured 8-inch cake pan.

Sift together the flour, carob or cocoa powder, sugar, salt, and
baking soda directly into the cake pan. Add the butter or margarine or oil, vinegar, vanilla, and water, and mix only until the larger
lumps are dissolved.

Bake for 30 minutes or until an inserted toothpick comes out
clean.

Cool, frost if desired, and serve.

Banana-Chocolate Frosting

Will frost one 8-inch completely cooled cake

1 cup butter *or* margarine *or* soft tofu

2 tablespoons carob powder *or* cocoa powder

1 large banana, peeled

1 tablespoon honey

Place all ingredients in food processor or blender; puree until smooth.

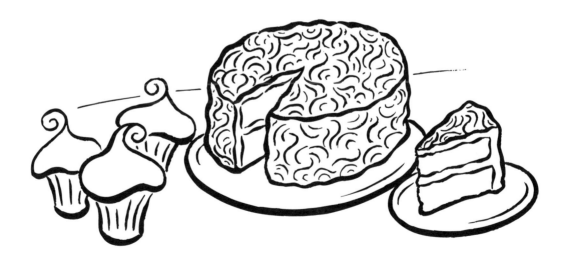

Cream Cheese Frosting

Will frost one 8-inch completely cooled cake

8 ounces dairy or nondairy cream cheese, softened

½ cup or more confectioners' sugar, to taste

1 teaspoon vanilla extract

In a medium bowl, beat confectioners' sugar and vanilla into the cream cheese. To make your own confectioners' sugar see page 11. Taste; if it's not sweet enough, add more confectioners' sugar, 1 tablespoon at a time.

Magic Frosting

This frosting can be made in many different colors and flavors.

Will frost one 8-inch cake

¼ cup margarine *or* butter *or* shortening

¼ cup honey *or* maple syrup

2–3 tablespoons rice milk *or* soy milk *or* cow's milk *or* fruit juice*

1 teaspoon any flavoring extract: vanilla, lemon, mint, rum, etc.

⅔ cup Better Than Milk powder *or* goat's-milk powder *or* soy-milk powder, unreconstituted

Fruit juice of your choice for color (optional)

Carob powder *or* cocoa powder (optional)

*Note: You may substitute a fruit juice in place of the milk; however, a very acidic juice like orange or pineapple will not work well. Try using apple juice, pear juice, or peach nectar.

Cream together margarine or butter or shortening and honey or maple syrup. Beat in milk or juice and your chosen flavoring extract. Add your selected milk powder, and continue beating until the frosting is light and fluffy. At this point, if the frosting is still too stiff, add more milk, little by little, to achieve the desired consistency.

Variation: Color may be created by adding a little cranberry juice for a pink frosting or a little purple grape juice for a lavender frosting. A chocolate flavor may be achieved by creaming in ¼ cup carob powder or cocoa powder immediately after adding the milk. Taste for desired sweetness. This will not work well, however, if you are using a fruit juice in place of the milk.

OTHER TOPPING
IDEAS

Sliced fresh seasonal fruits or berries will always dress up the plainest cakes.

Jams and jellies (corn syrup-free) can be spread between cooled cake layers or drizzled on the top of a still-hot cake to make a fancy dessert. See Breakfast Ideas (chapter 9) for creating your own home-made jams and jellies.

Chocolate chips or carob chips may be melted in the microwave or on top of the stove in a small saucepan and quickly drizzled over the top of your cake or cupcakes.

Chocolate candy bars or chocolate chips or carob chips may be placed on top of a completely baked cake, which is then returned to the oven, now turned off, for several minutes to allow the chocolate or carob to melt.

A nondairy whipped topping is delightful for cooled cakes or cupcakes.

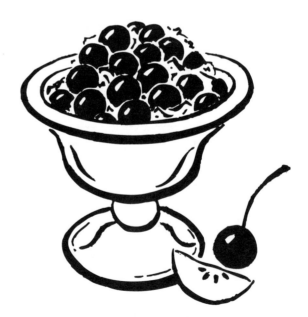

4

Berry and Fruit Delights

T he variety of fruit and berry desserts across our country is amazing. Some of our favorite regional recipes were carried across the ocean by colonists and immigrants, then modified to suit the fruits and berries available in the New World.

To peel or not to peel, that is the question. We feel it's a personal choice. Nutrients and fiber are lost when the peel is discarded; however, purists feel that the peel does not bake well. Do whatever you prefer. If you want to peel soft skinned fruit, simply dip them into boiling water for 30 seconds, then remove with a slotted spoon, and plunge them into ice water. Slip off the peels.

Some fruits adapt well to any recipe, while some are too dry or too juicy to substitute easily. Varieties of pears, for example, may differ greatly in appearance, but are very similar in cooking and baking qualities. Apple varieties, however, differ greatly. Red Delicious and Gala apples do not cook well in pies; all remaining varieties, such as Paula Red, Empire, McIntosh, Golden Delicious, IdaRed, Jonathan, Granny Smith, and Jonagold, will bake nicely. Rome Beauty and Northern Spy are a little too tart to eat fresh, but cook up well. According to the Michigan Apple Committee, three medium-sized fresh apples weigh approximately one pound, and six to eight medium-sized fresh apples will yield one nine-inch pie. Fresh blueberries may be stored in the refrigerator for up to fourteen days if covered. To freeze berries, sort and rinse them and allow them to dry, then freeze them in a single layer in a baking dish. Once frozen, they may be stored in the freezer in airtight containers for up to two years. Either fresh or frozen fruits and berries may be used in any of these recipes. An important tip—whenever berries are used in a dough or batter, coat them first in a separate

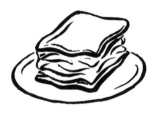

Buckle
Related to coffeecake. Fresh fruit is folded into a flour-and-butter batter, covered with a crunchy topping, and baked into a cakelike dessert.

Clafouti
Fruit is stirred into a custardy mixture and baked in a piecrust shell.

Cobbler
Sweetened, thickened fruit is covered with a biscuitlike crust and baked in a deep pan.

Crisp
Sweetened, thickened fruit is covered with a crunchy topping and baked in a deep pie pan or casserole dish.

Crumble

Flour and butter are cut together into a crumbly mixture, sprinkled on top of fruit, and baked in a pie pan.

Grunt

Flour and butter are blended and dropped by spoonfuls atop slightly sweetened fruit, then covered and steamed on the stovetop.

Slump

Sweetened fruit in a thickened sauce is covered with a soft flour-and-butter crust, then covered and steamed on the stovetop.

bowl with a little bit of the flour from the recipe. This will keep them from sinking into the dough or batter when baking.

Most of all, have fun! Try different seasonal fresh fruits and berries. Splurge on a package of frozen berries in the wintertime. Throw in a spice you haven't tried before, like fresh grated ginger with peaches, or cloves with pears. Remember, even if the appearance is a bit unusual, it will still taste great.

Because certain flours work best for crusts and toppings, you will find these recipes in their own chapter. Most of the toppings will be included with each recipe, but you can use a different one or create one of your own with a little guidance from chapter 6. The following chart describes some flours and their proportions that work well for the biscuit or dough toppings.

Dough Flour Chart

All combinations are for 1 cup.
NO means the flour alone or that combination of flours is not appropriate for a good dough topping.
OK means the flour may be used by itself and does not require another flour in addition to it.
ANY COMB. means any ratio of the two flours that adds up to 1 cup will make a good dough topping.

	Amaranth	Barley	Chickpea/Garbanzo	Millet	Oat
Amaranth	OK	1/3 cup barley with $^2/_3$ cup amaranth	up to 1/3 cup chickpea with $^2/_3$ cup or more amaranth	1/3 cup millet with $^2/_3$ cup amaranth	ANY COMB.
Barley	$^1/_3$ cup barley with $^2/_3$ cup amaranth	NO	NO	ANY COMB.	ANY COMB.
Chickpea/ Garbanzo	up to $^1/_3$ cup chickpea with $^2/_3$ cup or more amarath	NO	NO	NO	up to ¼ cup chickpea with ¾ cup or more oat

	Amaranth	Barley	Chickpea/Garbanzo	Millet	Oat
Millet	1/3 cup millet with 2/3 cup amaranth	ANY COMB.	NO	NO	ANY COMB.
Oat	ANY COMB.	ANY COMB.	up to ¼ cup chickpea with ¾ cup or more oat	ANY COMB.	OK
Potato	up to ¼ cup potato with ¾ cup or more amaranth	NO	NO	NO	up to ¼ cup potato with ¾ cup or more oat
Quinoa	ANY COMB.	¼ cup barley with ¾ cup quinoa	NO	NO	¼ cup quinoa with ¾ cup oat
Rice	NO	NO	NO	NO	¼ cup rice with ¾ cup oat
Soy	NO	NO	NO	NO	¼ cup soy with ¾ cup oat
Spelt	ANY COMB.	½ cup barley with ½ cup spelt	¼ cup chickpea with ¾ cup spelt	ANY COMB.	ANY COMB.

	Potato	Quinoa	Rice	Soy	Spelt
Amaranth	up to ¼ cup potato with ¾ cup or more amaranth	ANY COMB.	NO	NO	ANY COMB.
Barley	NO	¼ cup barley with ¾ cup quinoa	NO	NO	½ cup barley with ½ cup spelt
Chickpea/ Garbanzo	NO	NO	NO	NO	¼ cup chickpea with ¾ cup spelt
Millet	NO	NO	NO	NO	ANY COMB.
Oat	up to ¼ cup potato with ¾ cup or more oat	¼ cup quinoa with ¾ cup oat	¼ cup rice with ¾ cup oat	¼ cup soy with ¾ cup oat	ANY COMB.
Potato	NO	NO	NO	NO	¼ cup potato with ¾ cup spelt
Quinoa	NO	OK	NO	NO	ANY COMB.
Rice	NO	NO	NO	NO	¼ cup rice with ¾ cup spelt
Soy	NO	NO	NO	NO	¼ cup soy with ¾ cup spelt
Spelt	¼ cup potato with ¾ cup spelt	ANY COMB.	¼ cup rice with ¾ cup spelt	¼ cup soy with ¾ cup spelt	OK

Nectarine or Peach Buckle

Makes 4–6 servings

Batter Filling

¾ cup sugar

1 egg yolk

½ teaspoon ginger (optional)

¼ cup softened margarine *or* softened butter

½ cup cow's milk *or* soy milk *or* rice milk

2 cups plus 1 tablespoon flour (e.g., any one or combination of oat, amaranth, *or* spelt; *or* see chart, this chapter), divided

2 teaspoons baking powder

1 teaspoon salt

5–6 nectarines *or* peaches, sliced thin

Topping

½ cup sugar

⅓ cup flour (such as oat, spelt, *or* amaranth *or* see chart, chapter 6)

1 teaspoon cinnamon

¼ cup margarine *or* butter

Preheat oven to 375°F. Grease and flour one 1½-quart casserole dish.

For the batter: In a large bowl, beat sugar, egg yolk, ginger, and margarine or butter. Add milk and mix well for a smooth batter. Add 2 cups flour, baking powder, and salt, and mix well. Toss the peaches or nectarines in the remaining 1 tablespoon flour to keep them from sinking to the bottom of the batter. Fold floured fruit into batter slowly and pour into casserole dish.

For the topping: Mix sugar, flour, and cinnamon well in a small bowl. Using table knives or pastry cutter, cut the margarine or butter into the mixture until you have pea-sized crumbs. Sprinkle the topping onto the fruit batter.

Bake for 45–50 minutes or until a toothpick inserted into the topping comes out clean. Serve warm or cooled.

Blueberry Buckle

Makes 4–6 servings

Batter Filling

¾ cup sugar

1 egg yolk

¼ cup softened margarine *or* softened butter

½ cup cow's milk *or* soy milk *or* rice milk

2 cups plus 1 tablespoon flour (e.g., any one or combination of oat *or* spelt; *or* see chart, this chapter), divided

2 teaspoons baking powder

1 teaspoon salt

2 cups fresh or frozen blueberries

Topping

½ cup sugar

⅓ cup flour (any one or combination of oat *or* spelt; *or* see chart, chapter 6)

1 teaspoon cinnamon

¼ cup margarine *or* butter

Preheat oven to 375°F. Grease and flour one 1½-quart casserole dish.

For the batter: In a large bowl, combine sugar, egg yolk, and margarine or butter. Add milk and mix well for a smooth batter. Add 2 cups flour, baking powder, and salt, and mix well. Toss blueberries in remaining 1 tablespoon flour to keep them from sinking to the bottom of the batter. Fold floured blueberries into batter slowly and pour into casserole dish.

For the topping: Mix sugar, flour, and cinnamon well in a small bowl. Using table knives or a pastry cutter, cut the margarine or butter into the mixture until you have pea-sized crumbs. Sprinkle this mixture on top of the blueberry batter.

Bake for 45–50 minutes or until a toothpick inserted into the topping comes out clean. Serve warm or cooled.

Apple Clafouti

Makes 4–6 servings

8 tablespoons butter *or* margarine, divided

3 large apples, peeled, cored, and thickly sliced

²/₃ cup sugar, divided

¼ cup dark rum (a sugar cane product) *or* cognac (a grape product)

½ teaspoon cinnamon

1 cup cow's milk *or* soy milk *or* rice milk

4½ tablespoons Ener-G Egg Replacer powder

1 tablespoon vanilla extract

½ cup oat flour

1 pinch salt

Preheat oven to 350°F. Use 1 tablespoon of the butter or margarine to grease one 1½-quart casserole dish.

Melt the remaining 7 tablespoons of butter or margarine in a large skillet. Add apples and cook slowly, stirring occasionally, until apples have become browned, approximately 10–12 minutes. Add ¹/₃ cup of the sugar, rum or cognac, and cinnamon. Mix well for 1 minute, then remove from heat and let stand for 15 minutes.

In a blender, combine milk, Ener-G Egg Replacer powder, and vanilla and blend well. Add flour, salt, and remaining ¹/₃ cup of sugar and blend well. Pour apple mixture into casserole dish. Pour batter over apples.

Bake 45 minutes or until batter has puffed up and turned golden. Serve warm.

Quick Cherry Clafouti

Makes 4–6 servings

¼ cup cow's milk *or* soy milk *or* rice milk

²/₃ cup sugar, divided

4½ tablespoons Ener-G Egg Replacer powder

1 tablespoon vanilla extract

⅛ teaspoon salt

²/₃ cup flour (e.g., any one or combination of oat *or* spelt; *or* see chart, this chapter)

3 cups fresh or thawed sweet or tart cherries, rinsed and pitted

Preheat oven to 350°F. Grease one 1½-quart casserole dish.

In a blender, put milk, ¹/₃ cup of the sugar, Ener-G Egg Replacer powder, vanilla, salt, and flour; blend at high speed for 1 minute. Pour some of the batter into the casserole dish until it is ¼ inch deep; bake 1–2 minutes, or until batter has slightly set. Spread the cherries over the partially baked batter and sprinkle with the remaining ¹/₃ cup sugar. Pour remaining batter over the cherries, smoothing batter with the back of a spoon if necessary.

Bake for 60 minutes or until an inserted toothpick comes out clean. Serve warm or cold.

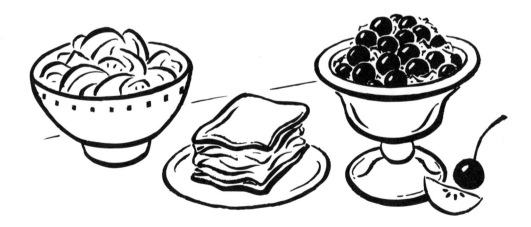

Blueberry Cobbler

Makes 4–6 servings

Filling

2 pints blueberries, washed

¼ cup sugar

2 tablespoons arrowroot flour *or* potato starch

1 tablespoon melted margarine *or* melted butter

1 tablespoon lemon juice

1 teaspoon grated lemon peel

⅛ teaspoon ground cloves

Batter

¼ cup sugar

¾ cup flour (e.g., any one or combination of oat *or* spelt; *or* see chart, this chapter)

¾ teaspoon baking powder

¼ teaspoon salt

1 egg yolk *or* 3 teaspoons Ener-G Egg Replacer powder

2 tablespoons cow's milk *or* soy milk *or* rice milk

2 tablespoons melted margarine *or* melted butter

Preheat oven to 400°F. Grease one 1½-quart casserole dish.

For the filling: In the casserole dish, mix berries, sugar, arrowroot flour or potato starch, margarine or butter, lemon juice, lemon peel, and cloves and set aside.

For the batter: In a separate medium bowl, mix sugar, flour, baking powder, and salt. Stir in egg yolk or Ener-G Egg Replacer powder, milk, and margarine or butter until a soft dough forms. If the dough seems too stiff, add another tablespoon of milk. Drop the dough by spoonfuls on top of the blueberry mixture.

Bake 30–35 minutes or until filling begins to bubble and crust is golden brown. Serve warm or cool.

Cranberry-Pear Cobbler

Makes 4–6 servings

Filling

1 tablespoon margarine *or* butter

5 medium pears, peeled, cored, and cut into ½-inch pieces

1 cup fresh or frozen cranberries

⅓ cup light or dark brown sugar, packed

⅓ cup sugar

3 tablespoons arrowroot flour

2 tablespoons lemon juice

2 teaspoons cinnamon

½ teaspoon ginger

Topping

1 cup flour (e.g., ½ cup oat and ½ cup barley; *or* see chart, chapter 6)

¼ cup sugar

1 teaspoon baking powder

½ tablespoon Ener-G Egg Replacer powder

2 tablespoons cold cow's milk *or* cold soy milk *or* ice water

¼ cup melted margarine *or* melted butter *or* mild-tasting oil

Preheat oven to 325°F. Use one ungreased 1½-quart casserole dish.

For the filling: In a large frying pan, melt the butter. Add pears and cook over low flame until soft. Remove pan from heat and stir in cranberries, brown sugar, sugar, arrowroot flour, lemon juice, cinnamon, and ginger. Mix well. Pour into casserole dish and set aside.

For the topping: In a separate medium bowl mix flour, sugar, baking powder, and Ener-G Egg Replacer powder. Add milk or ice water and stir only until combined. Fold in margarine or butter or oil. Spoon topping evenly over filling.

Bake 55–60 minutes, or until topping is browned and filling is bubbly. Serve warm or cold.

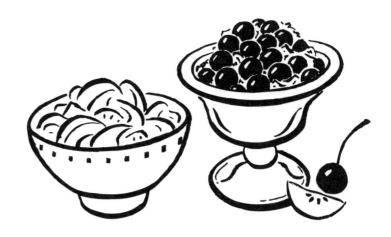

Microwave Berry Cobbler

Makes 6 servings

Filling

4 cups berries (all one kind or mixed, *or* try 1 cup diced peaches with 3 cups berries*)

4 tablespoons sugar

2 tablespoons arrowroot flour *or* potato starch

1 teaspoon lemon juice

½ teaspoon grated lemon peel

Batter

½ cup flour (e.g., any one or combination of oat *or* spelt; *or* see chart, this chapter)

1 tablespoon sugar

¼ teaspoon baking soda

1/8 teaspoon nutmeg

2 tablespoons dairy or nondairy yogurt

2 tablespoons melted butter *or* melted margarine *or* mild-tasting oil

Topping

1 tablespoon sugar

1/8 teaspoon cinnamon

For the filling: In a 1½-quart microwave-safe casserole dish, combine fruit, sugar, arrowroot flour or potato starch, lemon juice, and lemon peel; microwave on HIGH for 6–7 minutes or until it begins to bubble and thicken. Rotate and stir halfway through cooking. Let filling cool in the casserole dish for 20–30 minutes to allow it to finish thickening.

For the batter: In a separate medium bowl, mix flour, sugar, baking soda, and nutmeg. Add yogurt and butter or margarine or oil and stir just until mixed. Divide dough into 6 equal balls, pat balls into ½-inch thick biscuits, put in a separate 1½-quart microwave-safe dish, and set aside.

For the topping: In a separate small bowl, mix sugar and cinnamon; sprinkle the topping evenly over the biscuits.

Microwave the biscuits with the topping on HIGH for 2–3 minutes or until centers spring back when gently touched.

To serve, rewarm the filling and ladle over the biscuits.

---

*Note that if you are using peaches, try adding 1 teaspoon grated fresh ginger to really snap up that peach taste. Also, microwave the filling for an additional 4–5 minutes, as peaches are juicier and will take longer to cook and thicken.

Peach Cobbler

Makes 6–8 servings

Filling

8 large peaches, sliced

3 tablespoons sugar

3 tablespoons bourbon (a corn product) *or* rum (a sugar cane product)

2 tablespoons butter *or* margarine

Batter

½ cup flour (e.g., any one or combination of oat *or* spelt; *or* see chart, this chapter)

2½ teaspoons baking powder

½ teaspoon salt

8 tablespoons margarine *or* butter

⅓ cup cow's milk *or* soy milk *or* rice milk

5 tablespoons sugar

Preheat oven to 425°F. Grease one 2½-quart casserole dish.

For the filling: Place sliced peaches in casserole dish. Sprinkle with sugar and the bourbon or rum; dot with the butter or margarine cut into small pieces.

For the batter: In a separate small bowl, mix flour, baking powder, and salt. Using table knives or a pastry cutter, cut the margarine or butter into the flour until the mixture is coarse and crumbly. Add milk and mix well until batter is very soft but not runny. If the batter still looks and feels stiff, add extra milk by teaspoonfuls until the batter consistency is very soft but not runny. Drop the batter in clumps over the peaches and refrigerate for 30 minutes. Remove from refrigerator, sprinkle 5 tablespoons sugar over the batter.

Bake for 30 minutes or until the batter is puffy and golden brown. Serve warm.

Apple Crisp

Serve this warm for a great winter dessert!

Makes one 9-inch crisp

Filling

6 cups tart apples, peeled and sliced thin

¼ cup chopped pecans, (optional)

¼ cup raisins

¹⁄₃ cup light or dark brown sugar, packed

Topping

¹⁄₃ cup light or dark brown sugar, packed

¹⁄₃ cup flour (e.g., oat *or* spelt; *or* see chart, chapter 6)

¹⁄₃ cup quick oats

½ teaspoon cinnamon

¼ teaspoon nutmeg

3 tablespoons butter *or* margarine

Preheat oven to 375°F. Use one ungreased 9-inch pie pan.

For the filling: Combine apples, pecans, and raisins in a large bowl. Place half this mixture in the pie pan. Sprinkle ¹⁄₃ cup brown sugar over the fruit in the pie pan and top with the remaining half of the mixture.

For the topping: In a separate medium bowl, combine ¹⁄₃ cup brown sugar, flour, oats, cinnamon, and nutmeg, mixing well. Using two table knives or a pastry cutter, cut in the butter or margarine until the mixture is coarse and crumbly. Sprinkle this topping over the fruit mixture.

Bake for 30–35 minutes or until the apples are tender when a fork or toothpick is inserted.

Apricot-Ginger Crisp

Makes 4–6 servings

Filling

⅓ cup light brown sugar, packed

3 tablespoons flour (e.g., oat *or* spelt; *or* see chart, this chapter)

¼ cup peeled and grated fresh ginger

1 teaspoon cinnamon

Grated peel of 1 lemon

2½ pounds fresh apricots, pitted and halved (approximately 5 cups)

Topping

¾ cup flour (e.g., oat *or* spelt; *or* see chart, chapter 6)

⅔ cup dark brown sugar, packed

¼ teaspoon salt

¼ teaspoon cinnamon

½ teaspoon ground ginger

6 tablespoons cold margarine *or* cold butter

Preheat oven to 375°F. Use one 1½-quart casserole dish.

For the filling: In a medium bowl, mix light brown sugar, flour, fresh ginger, cinnamon, and lemon peel. Add apricots; thoroughly toss to coat fruit, and place in casserole dish.

For the topping: In a separate medium bowl, combine flour, dark brown sugar, salt, cinnamon, and ground ginger. Using two table knives or a pastry cutter, cut in the margarine or butter until the mixture is coarse and crumbly.

Cover the filling evenly with the topping.

Bake 20–30 minutes or until the apricots have softened and topping is golden brown. Serve warm.

Microwave Peach Crisp

Makes 4–6 servings

Filling

2 pounds peaches, pitted and sliced

2 tablespoons light or dark brown sugar, packed

Topping

8 cinnamon *or* gingersnap cookies (see chapter 7 for recipe)

2 tablespoons chopped walnuts

2 teaspoons mild-tasting oil

For the filling: In a 1½-quart microwave-safe casserole dish, combine peaches and brown sugar.

For the topping: Place cookies in a plastic bag. Using a rolling pin or hammer, crush cookies. Add the walnuts to the crushed cookie mixture and shake to mix well. Add oil to the nut and cookie mixture and knead bag to mix well. Sprinkle this topping over the peaches.

Microwave loosely covered on HIGH for 3 minutes. Uncover the dish, rotate, and microwave on HIGH for another 2 minutes. Cool for 20–25 minutes before serving.

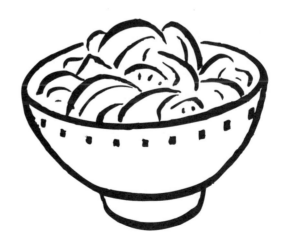

Peach Crisp

Filling

5 large peaches, pitted and sliced

1 tablespoon maple syrup *or* honey

1 tablespoon lemon juice

1 tablespoon oat flour

Topping

1 tablespoon oat flour

½ cup quick oats

¼ teaspoon salt

4 tablespoons maple syrup *or* honey

1 tablespoon mild-tasting oil

1 tablespoon butter *or* margarine

1 teaspoon vanilla extract

Preheat oven to 375°F. Use one 1½-quart casserole dish.

For the filling: In a medium bowl, toss the peaches with the maple syrup or honey, lemon juice, and flour, and spread evenly into casserole dish.

For the topping: In a separate small bowl, mix the flour, quick oats, and salt. In another small bowl, cream together the maple syrup or honey, oil, butter or margarine, and vanilla. To this mixture, add the flour, oat, and salt mixture; mix well and sprinkle evenly over the peach filling.

Bake for 20–25 minutes, until peaches are bubbling and topping begins to brown.

Variation: Try 1½ cups granola (see chapter 9 for recipe) instead of the topping.

Microwave Plum Crumble

Makes 4–6 servings

Filling

4 medium plums, pitted and sliced

2 tablespoons honey

2 tablespoons arrowroot flour *or* potato starch

Topping

3 tablespoons quick oats

3 tablespoons light or dark brown sugar, packed

2 teaspoons oat flour

¼ teaspoon cinnamon

1/8 teaspoon nutmeg

1 tablespoon butter *or* margarine

For the filling: In a 1½-quart microwave-safe casserole dish, combine plums, honey, and arrowroot flour or potato starch.

For the topping: In a small bowl combine quick oats, brown sugar, flour, cinnamon, and nutmeg. Using two table knives or a pastry cutter, cut the butter or margarine into the mixture until coarse and crumbly. Sprinkle evenly over the filling.

Microwave on HIGH for 6–7 minutes or until filling begins to bubble; rotate midway through cooking. Cool 20–30 minutes before serving.

Rhubarb-Strawberry Crumble

Makes 4–6 servings

Filling

1 pound rhubarb, cleaned and cut in ¼-inch pieces

1 pint strawberries, hulled and halved

¾ cup sugar

Grated peel of 1 orange

¼ cup orange juice

3 tablespoons arrowroot flour *or* kudzu powder

Topping

1 cup quick oats

⅓ cup oat flour

¼ cup light brown sugar, packed

½ teaspoon cinnamon

½ cup chopped pecans *or* walnuts (optional)

5 tablespoons cold margarine *or* cold butter

Preheat oven to 350°F. Grease one 8-inch nonaluminum cake pan or baking dish.

For the filling: In a large bowl, mix rhubarb, strawberries, sugar, orange peel, orange juice, and arrowroot flour or kudzu powder. Pour mixture into baking dish.

For the topping: In a small bowl, mix quick oats, flour, brown sugar, cinnamon, and nuts. Using two table knives or a pastry cutter, cut margarine or butter into mixture until coarse and crumbly. Sprinkle over filling.

Bake for 45–50 minutes, until the fruit filling in the middle of the baking dish is thick and clear. Serve warm or cool.

Blueberry Grunt

Makes 6–8 servings

Filling

6 cups blueberries, rinsed

1 cup water

1 cup sugar

1 teaspoon arrowroot flour

½ teaspoon cinnamon

Dough

1¾ cups flour (e.g., 1 ¼ cups oat *or* spelt and ½ cup millet *or* barley; *or* see chart, this chapter)

½ teaspoon salt

1 tablespoon baking powder

6 tablespoons cold margarine *or* cold butter

¾ cup cow's milk *or* soy milk *or* rice milk

For the filling: In a large saucepan or a deep skillet, mix blueberries, water, sugar, arrowroot flour, and cinnamon. On top of the stove over a high heat, bring the berry filling to a boil, then simmer on low heat for 10 minutes, until the berries begin to soften.

For the dough: In a medium bowl, mix flour, salt, and baking powder well. Using two table knives or a pastry cutter, cut in margarine or butter until dough is coarse and crumbly. Add milk and mix just well enough to combine into a soft dough. Drop the dough by tablespoonfuls onto the berry filling mixture, then turn up the heat slightly so that berry mixture bubbles slowly; cover the saucepan or skillet.

Cook for 15–20 minutes, until the dough has formed cooked dumplings. (A dumpling is cooked when it has lost its raw, almost shiny look, and steam rises when the dumpling is pierced with a fork.)

Place the dumplings in individual serving bowls and cover with the berry filling. Serve hot or warm.

New England Berry Grunt

Makes 4 servings

Filling

1 pint berries, any type, rinsed

1 cup water

½ cup sugar

Dough

½ cup flour (e.g., oat *or* spelt; *or* see chart, this chapter)

1 tablespoon baking powder

¼ teaspoon salt

1 tablespoon chilled margarine *or* chilled butter

¼ cup cow's milk *or* soy milk *or* goat's milk *or* almond milk

For the filling: In a medium saucepan, combine the berries, water, and sugar. Cook over low heat until the berries soften, approximately 8–10 minutes.

For the dough: In a small bowl, mix flour, baking powder, and salt. Using two table knives or a pastry cutter, cut in margarine or butter until the dough is coarse and crumbly. Add milk and mix to form a soft dough.

Pour the berry filling into a 1½-quart round casserole dish, and drop the dough by large spoonfuls on top of the filling. Cover the dish with a lid or foil and place inside a deep pot on top of your stove. Pour enough water into the pot to reach halfway up the side of the dish and simmer on low heat for 30 minutes, or until the dough has formed soft, cooked dumplings. (A dumpling is cooked when it has lost its raw, almost shiny look, and steam rises when the dumpling is pierced with a fork.) Check the water level periodically and replace with boiling water if evaporating. Serve hot.

Apple Pandowdy

Makes 6–8 servings

Filling

6 medium apples, peeled and sliced

½ cup sugar

½ teaspoon cinnamon

¼ teaspoon salt

¼ teaspoon nutmeg

½ cup maple syrup

3 tablespoons water

2 tablespoons melted butter *or* melted margarine *or* mild-tasting oil

Dough

1 cup flour (e.g., ½ cup oat and ½ cup barley; *or* see chart, this chapter)

2 tablespoons sugar

¼ teaspoon salt

^{1}/₃ cup shortening *or* butter *or* margarine *or* mild-tasting oil

3 tablespoons cold cow's milk *or* ice water *or* cold soy milk *or* cold rice milk

2 tablespoons melted butter *or* melted margarine *or* mild-tasting oil

Preheat oven to 350°F. Use one ungreased 2½-quart casserole dish.

For the filling: In a large bowl, mix apples, sugar, cinnamon, salt, and nutmeg. Place into casserole dish. In a separate bowl, mix maple syrup, water, and melted butter or melted margarine or oil. Pour over apple mixture.

For the dough: In a separate medium bowl, mix flour, sugar, and salt. Using two table knives or a pastry cutter, cut in shortening or butter or margarine or oil into flour mixture. Sprinkle in milk or ice water one tablespoonful at a time and knead until well mixed (the dough should clean off the sides of the bowl when rolled around). Shape the dough into a ball and place on a lightly floured surface. Roll out to fit snugly into the casserole dish.

Place the dough over the apple mixture and lightly brush the top of the dough with 2 tablespoons melted butter or melted margarine or oil.

Bake for 30 minutes. Remove dish from oven and, using a sharp knife, cut the crust into small pieces, gently mixing the pieces into the apple filling. Return to oven and bake another 30–45 minutes or until apples are tender and crust pieces are golden brown. Serve hot or cold.

Blueberry Slump

Dough

1 cup flour (e.g., ½ cup oat and ½ cup barley; *or* see chart, this chapter)

1 tablespoon sugar

1 teaspoon baking powder

½ teaspoon salt

1 egg yolk *or* ½ teaspoon Ener-G Egg Replacer powder

3 tablespoons cow's milk *or* soy milk *or* rice milk

2 tablespoons melted margarine *or* melted butter

Filling

1 quart blueberries, rinsed

½ cup sugar

½ cup water

½ teaspoon nutmeg

For the dough: In a large bowl, mix flour, sugar, baking powder, and salt. Stir in egg yolk or Ener-G Egg Replacer powder and mix well. Add milk and margarine or butter, stirring to form a soft dough.

For the filling: In a medium saucepan, heat the blueberries, sugar, water, and nutmeg over high heat on top of the stove until the filling is boiling. Continue boiling and stirring until the filling is almost a sauce, approximately 10 minutes. Reduce heat to medium.

Using a large spoon, drop the dough onto the blueberry filling. Cover the saucepan and leave over medium heat until the dough has formed soft, cooked dumplings, about 10 minutes. (A dumpling is cooked when it has lost its raw, almost shiny look, and steam rises when the dumpling is pierced with a fork.)

Spoon the cooked dumplings into serving bowls and ladle the blueberry filling over them. Serve warm.

5 Humble Pie and the Queen of Tarts

What would childhood and summer be like without a pie cooling in the kitchen? Or Thanksgiving without an apple or pumpkin pie for dessert? Pies are truly an American favorite and not tied to any particular season. They are relatively easy to make and use fewer ingredients than most other desserts. You can use whatever fruits you have available. Though fresh seasonal fruits are always best, frozen, canned, or dried fruits work well, too. The combinations of flavors and choices are endless and your family will welcome these satisfying desserts year-round.

Once you have explored the recipes in this chapter, you may be inspired to develop a few fillings uniquely your own. Enjoy!

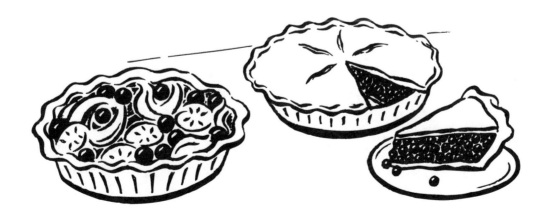

Deep-Dish Apple-Rhubarb Pie

*Makes one 10-inch
deep-dish pie*

Crust

Dough for two 9-inch
piecrusts rolled out to 18
inches across (the pastry
crust works best with this
pie; see chapter 6 for
recipe)

Filling

¼ cup sugar

¼ cup arrowroot flour

1 teaspoon cinnamon

4 large Granny Smith apples,
cored and sliced into small
wedges

2 tablespoons margarine *or*
butter

1 tablespoon lemon juice

2 pounds rhubarb stalks,
cleaned and chopped into 1-
inch pieces

Prepare the pie dough according to directions. Roll out and set aside.

Preheat oven to 400°F. Use one 2½-quart square casserole dish. *For the filling*: In a large nonaluminum saucepan, combine sugar, arrowroot flour, and cinnamon until well mixed. Stir in apples, butter or margarine, and lemon juice; let sit for 5 minutes. Cover and cook over low heat on top of the stove until the apples begin to soften and the sauce begins to bubble, stirring occasionally. Remove from heat and stir in the rhubarb. Cool filling to room temperature.

Line the dish with the rolled-out dough, leaving dough hanging out over the rim. Mound the filling into the center, and bring the overhanging edges toward the middle of the filling, forming the dough into pleats or folds to allow it to lay flat on top of the filling. The center of the filling will be uncovered.

Place the casserole dish on a cookie sheet to catch drips as the pie bakes, and bake for 25 minutes. Lower the oven temperature to 350°F, cover the pie with aluminum foil, and bake another 25–35 minutes, or until the filling begins to bubble at the center. Cool and serve.

Banana Cream Pie

Crust

1 fully baked 9-inch piecrust
(use your favorite; see
chapter 6 for recipes)

Filling

½ cup sugar, divided
5 tablespoons oat flour
½ teaspoon salt
2½ cups cow's milk *or* rice
milk *or* soy milk
3 egg yolks
1 teaspoon vanilla extract
3 bananas, sliced

Prepare and bake the piecrust according to directions; set aside.

For the filling: Mix ¼ cup sugar, flour, and salt in the top of a double boiler. Add milk and cook over a medium heat, stirring constantly until all of the sugar and salt have dissolved. Cover and let cook for 15 minutes more, stirring occasionally.

In a separate bowl, beat the egg yolks with the remaining ¼ cup sugar until creamy. Stir a little hot filling mixture from the double boiler into the yolk and sugar mixture to warm it. Add the yolk and sugar mixture to the filling mixture in the double boiler and cook for 2 more minutes over a medium heat, stirring constantly. Remove from heat and cool to room temperature.

When the filling has cooled, add the vanilla and stir in well. Spoon a thin layer of the filling into the baked piecrust. Top with a layer of sliced bananas. Spoon on another layer of filling, and add another layer of sliced bananas. Continue until all the filling and bananas are used. Chill in the refrigerator for at least one hour before serving.

Serve with whipped topping if desired.

Blueberry Pie

Makes one 9-inch pie

Crust

Dough for one 9-inch piecrust (use your favorite; see chapter 6 for recipes)

Filling

2 pints blueberries, rinsed

$1/3$ cup margarine *or* butter

1 cup dark brown sugar, packed

$1/2$ teaspoon cinnamon

Grated peel of 1 lemon

$1/2$ cup lemon juice

$1/3$ cup arrowroot flour *or* kudzu powder

Prepare the pie dough according to directions. Roll out.

Preheat oven to 400°F. Line one ungreased 9-inch pie pan with rolled-out pie dough.

For the filling: In a medium saucepan, mix the blueberries, margarine or butter, brown sugar, cinnamon, and lemon peel. Heat on top of the stove over medium heat, stirring constantly, until the berries are softened, approximately 5 minutes. In a small bowl, mix the lemon juice and arrowroot flour or kudzu powder until all lumps are dissolved. Add to the berry filling in the saucepan and stir over low to medium heat until the filling begins to thicken.

Remove the saucepan from heat and let the filling cool. When cooled, pour filling into the unbaked crust.

Place the pie pan on a cookie sheet to catch any drips and bake for 45 minutes or until filling is bubbling. Serve warm or cool.

Cherry Pie

Makes one 9-inch pie

Crust

Dough for one 9-inch piecrust, *or* double the recipe if you want a top crust (use your favorite; see chapter 6 for recipes)

Filling

4 cups tart cherries, rinsed and pitted

$1/3$ cup sugar

2 tablespoons plus 2 teaspoons quick-cooking tapioca

2 tablespoons kirsch (cherry brandy liqueur, optional)

2 tablespoons chilled margarine *or* chilled butter

Prepare the pie dough according to directions. Roll out.

Preheat oven to 450°F. Line one 9-inch pie pan with rolled-out dough.

For the filling: Mix cherries, sugar, tapioca, and kirsch; let stand for 15 minutes. Pour fruit into unbaked piecrust and dot with margarine or butter. If you are using a top crust, put it on over the filling. Be sure to score the edges to seal it and cut slits in the top to allow steam to escape.

Bake for 10 minutes, then reduce oven temperature to 350°F and continue baking another 40 minutes, until the edges of the crust are golden brown. Cool and serve.

Nectarine Crumble Pie

Makes one 9-inch pie

Crust

1 fully baked 9-inch piecrust (use your favorite; see chapter 6 for recipes)

Filling

3 pounds ripe nectarines, sliced

2/3 cup sugar

1/4 cup any flour containing gluten (such as oat *or* barley; *or* see chart, chapter 1)

3 tablespoons lemon juice

1/4 teaspoon almond extract *or* vanilla extract

Topping

2/3 cup flour (e.g., oat *or* spelt; *or* see chart, chapter 6)

1/2 cup sugar

1/2 cup chilled margarine *or* chilled butter

Prepare and bake the piecrust according to directions; set aside. Preheat oven to 450°F.

For the filling: In a large bowl, mix nectarines, sugar, flour, lemon juice, and almond or vanilla extract, tossing well to completely coat the fruit. Spoon into cooked piecrust.

For the topping: In a separate small bowl mix flour and sugar. Using two table knives or a pastry cutter, cut the margarine or butter into the mixture until mixture is coarse and crumbly. Sprinkle over the filling.

Bake for 15 minutes at 450°F; then reduce oven temperature to 350°F and bake for another 40–45 minutes. Cool and serve.

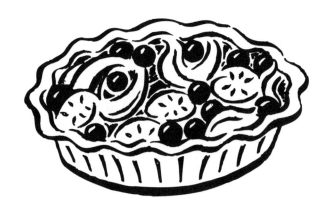

Shoofly Pie

Makes one 9-inch pie

Crust

Dough for one 9-inch piecrust (use your favorite; see chapter 6 for recipes)

Filling

½ cup any flour containing gluten (such as oat *or* amaranth; *or* see chart; chapter 1)

1 cup light or dark brown sugar, packed

$\frac{1}{8}$ teaspoon salt

4 tablespoons cold butter *or* cold margarine

2 teaspoons baking soda

½ cup light molasses

Prepare the pie dough according to directions. Roll out.

Preheat oven to 350°F. Line one 9-inch pie pan with rolled-out dough.

Combine flour, brown sugar, salt, and butter or margarine. Mix only until crumbly; do not overmix. In a small saucepan, dissolve the baking soda and molasses on top of the stove over a very low heat. Add ¾ of the crumbly mixture to the saucepan and mix well. Pour this into the pie pan. Sprinkle the remaining ¼ of the crumbly mixture over the top.

Bake for 30 minutes or until the center is firm. Serve slightly warm or cold.

Very Berry Pie

Makes one 9-inch pie

Crust

Dough for two 9-inch pie pans (the dough crust works best; see chapter 6 for recipe)

Filling

9 cups mixed berries, any combination*

1 tablespoon lemon juice

1 tablespoon any mild-tasting flour (such as oat, barley, millet, *or* soy)

$2/3$–1 cup sugar, to taste

¼ cup quick-cooking small pearl tapioca

1 pinch salt

2 tablespoons chilled margarine *or* chilled butter

---

*Note that 4 cups of mixed berries makes a delicious but much lower pie if you don't have 9 cups of berries on hand; just reduce the sugar to $1/3$ cup.

Prepare the pie dough according to directions. Roll out.

Preheat oven to 400°F. Line one 9-inch pie pan with rolled-out dough and reserve second dough for the top crust.

For the filling: Toss berries with lemon juice, flour, sugar, tapioca, and salt. Let stand for 20 minutes. Place the berry filling in the pie pan and dot with margarine or butter. Place the second crust on top, crimping the edges to seal; cut slits in the top to allow steam to escape.

Bake approximately 45 minutes or until the crust is deep brown and the filling is bubbly. Let the pie cool at least 2 hours to allow the juices to thicken before serving.

To serve slightly warm, reheat in oven at 300°F for 15 minutes.

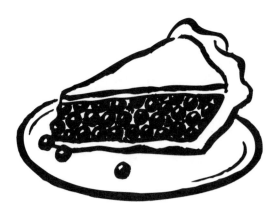

Vinegar Pie

Makes one 9-inch pie

Crust

1 fully baked 9-inch piecrust (the dough crust works best; see chapter 6 for recipe)

Filling

8 tablespoons margarine *or* butter

2 tablespoons any mild-tasting flour (such as oat, barley, millet, *or* soy)

1 cup dark brown sugar, packed

½ cup sugar

4 egg yolks *or* 4½ teaspoons Ener-G Egg Replacer powder

¼ cup apple juice

¼ cup cider vinegar

¼ cup chopped walnuts *or* pecans (optional)

Prepare and bake the piecrust according to directions; set aside.

Preheat oven to 375°F.

For the filling: In a medium bowl, cream together the margarine or butter, flour, brown sugar, and sugar. Add the egg yolks or Ener-G Egg Replacer powder and beat until fluffy. Stir in apple juice and vinegar until blended. Pour into baked piecrust and sprinkle with chopped nuts.

Bake for 50–60 minutes or until an inserted toothpick comes out clean. Cool before serving.

Apple-Raisin Tart

Makes one 11-inch tart or one 9-inch pie

Crust

Dough for one 9-inch piecrust (use your favorite; see chapter 6 for recipes)

Filling

6 medium apples, peeled, cored, and sliced

1 tablespoon lemon juice

½ cup raisins

1 cup sugar

½ tablespoon any mild-tasting flour (such as soy, millet, barley, *or* oat)

1 teaspoon cinnamon

¼ teaspoon nutmeg

Prepare the pie dough according to directions. Roll out.

Preheat oven to 400°F. Line one 11-inch tart pan or one 9-inch pie pan with rolled-out dough.

For the filling: In a medium bowl, mix apples, lemon juice, and raisins well. Add sugar, flour, cinnamon, and nutmeg; combine well. Spread evenly over the dough.

Bake for 40–50 minutes, until the edges of the pastry are well browned and apple edges begin to brown. Cool slightly.

This may be served with a whipped topping.

Pear Tart

Makes 6 tarts

Crust

Dough for one 9-inch piecrust (use your favorite; see chapter 6 for recipes)

Filling

¼ cup margarine *or* butter

½ cup light or dark brown sugar, packed

1 tablespoon brandy *or* dark rum

1 teaspoon lemon juice

¼ teaspoon cinnamon

2 large pears, peeled, quartered, and cored

Prepare the pie dough according to directions. Roll out and set aside.

Preheat oven to 375°F. Use one large ungreased cookie sheet.

For the filling: In a large frying pan, melt margarine or butter over medium heat on top of the stove. Add the brown sugar, brandy or rum, lemon juice, and cinnamon; stir over medium heat until the sugar dissolves. Slice each pear quarter lengthwise into 4 even slices and add to the liquid in the frying pan. Poach the pear slices gently until tender, about 8–10 minutes.

Using a slotted spoon, remove the pear slices to a plate and set them aside. Heat the liquid in the frying pan over a high heat until it is reduced to a thick bubbling syrup, about 1 minute. Set aside.

Place the rolled-out pie dough on a lightly floured board. Using the tip of a sharp knife, cut out 6 pieces in the shape of whole pears, approximately 3" x 5" each. Place the pastry shapes on an ungreased cookie sheet. Arrange 5 pear slices on top of each shape, fanning pieces to resemble a whole pear, and leave a small border of pastry around slices. Fit the 2 remaining slices onto any two pastry shapes, or eat them. Brush the reduced syrup on top of the pear slices.

Bake 10–15 minutes or until pastry is golden brown. Serve warm or cooled.

6 Crusts and Toppings

S ome pastry chefs talk about kneading pie dough until the fat (butter, margarine, oil, or shortening) is well mixed into the flour. Some warn of dire consequences if the dough is kneaded or rolled even a moment longer than necessary. Some require ice water for a flaky crust; some use vinegar; some swear by lard; some will use only the best butter.

What works for you? Frankly, a crust, unless it is a thick pastry designed to be an integral part of the dessert, is only a thing to hold the fruit filling together until you eat it. Nice, easy to make, stable crusts for your favorite fillings follow.

A general topping is included, because recipes that include various specific toppings are found in chapter 4. We recommend that you jot down a list of topping ingredients that work well for you and add it to this chapter as your own.

We found an easy way to roll out a crust using plastic wrap: Take a sheet of plastic wrap a little larger than twice the size of the top of the pie pan. Place the dough ball in the center of one-half of the plastic wrap; fold the other half over the dough ball, also centering that half. Using a rolling pin, begin to roll out a circle of dough, periodically lifting and repositioning the plastic wrap to avoid "wrinkles" in your crust, turning the whole thing over, and rolling out the other side. When the dough has reached the desired thickness and circumference, simply peel back the upper layer of plastic wrap, slide your hand under the bottom layer, and turn the crust over into your pie pan. Use the plastic wrap to help you lift and tuck the dough completely into the pan and down its sides. Then peel the plastic wrap off the top of the dough and throw it away. No floury mess, no sticky dough on your roller, no counter to clean up!

A chart follows to help you select the flour or flour combinations that we have found work best for crusts and toppings.

Piecrust and Topping Flour Chart

These are suggested combinations of flours that work well for piecrusts. All combinations are for 1½ cups flour.

NO means the flour alone or that combination of flours is not appropriate for a good piecrust.

OK means the flour may be used by itself and does not require another flour in addition to it.

ANY COMB. means any ratio of the two flours that adds up to 1½ cups will make a good piecrust.

	Amaranth	Barley	Oat	Potato	Quinoa	Spelt
Amaranth	NO	NO	ANY COMB.	1¼ cup amaranth, ¼ cup potato	ANY COMB.	ANY COMB.
Barley	NO	NO	½ cup barley, 1 cup oat	NO	½ cup barley, 1 cup oat	½ cup barley, 1 cup oat
Oat	ANY COMB.	1 cup oat, ½ cup barley	OK	NO	ANY COMB.	ANY COMB.
Potato	¼ cup potato, 1¼ cup amaranth	NO	NO	NO	¼ cup potato, 1¼ cup quinoa	¼ cup potato, 1¼ cup spelt
Quinoa	ANY COMB.	1 cup quinoa, ½ cup barley	ANY COMB.	1¼ cup quinoa, ¼ cup potato	OK	ANY COMB.
Spelt	ANY COMB.	1 cup spelt, ½ cup barley	ANY COMB.	1¼ cup spelt, ¼ cup potato	ANY COMB.	OK

Coconut Crust

Makes one 9-inch crust

1 cup unsweetened shredded
coconut

2 tablespoons mild-tasting oil

2 tablespoons honey

Combine all ingredients. Press into 9-inch pie pan. Bake at 325°F for 5–8 minutes. Cool and fill with desired filling.

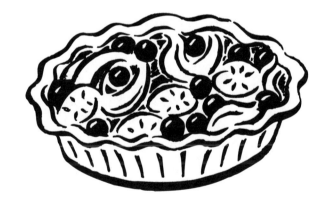

Dough Crust

1 cup oat flour
½ cup barley flour
½ teaspoon salt
4 tablespoons butter *or* margarine
1 tablespoon mild-tasting oil
4 tablespoons ice water

Sift together the flours and the salt. Knead or cut in the butter or margarine, then the oil, and gently knead in the water. Roll into a ball and flatten with your hands. Using a floured rolling pin, roll the dough out slowly until it is large enough to cover the bottom and sides of one 9-inch pie pan. Gently press the dough into the pie pan and bake at 325°F for 5-8 minutes, until edges begin to turn golden, or fill with filling and bake as directed.

Note that this recipe will give you enough dough to also make a thin top crust if you roll out a thinner ¼-inch bottom crust. You can roll out a very thin top crust, or use the dough for a lattice crust. For a sweeter crust, add 1 tablespoon confectioners' sugar (see chapter 2 for recipe) to the sifted flour and salt mixture, then proceed as above. Sometimes bakers use lard for a very flaky crust. If you don't mind using an animal fat, then lard is an acceptable substitute.

Granola Crust

Makes one 9-inch crust

½ cup granola (see chapter 9 for recipe)

2 tablespoons mild-tasting oil

2 tablespoons honey

Combine all ingredients. Press into 9-inch pie pan. Bake at 325°F for 5–8 minutes. Cool and fill with desired filling, then bake as directed.

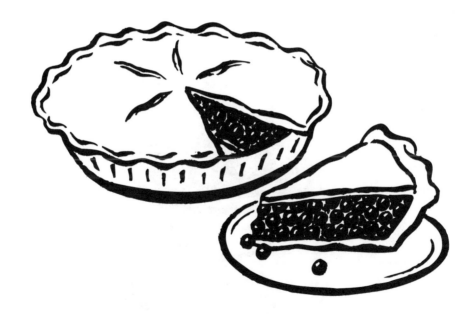

Cherry Compote

This is a great topping for ice cream or chocolate cake.

Makes approximately 4 cups

2 pounds fresh tart or sweet cherries, rinsed and pitted

¼ cup sugar

1 teaspoon kirsch (cherry brandy liqueur)

2–3 teaspoons balsamic vinegar

Place the cherries in a large skillet and sprinkle them with the sugar. Heat over high heat on top of the stove, shaking the pan often until the sugar melts and the cherries begin to feel soft. Add kirsch and vinegar and gently shake the pan for another 30 seconds. Place the compote in a large bowl and refrigerate for at least one hour before serving.

Serve over ice cream or with hard cookies.

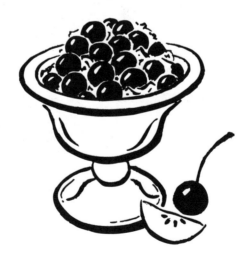

Streusel Topping

*Tops one 8-inch cake or
9-inch pie*

1/3 cup light or dark brown
  sugar, packed

2 tablespoons sugar

1½ teaspoons cinnamon

½ cup flour (e.g., oat, spelt,
  or amaranth; *or* see chart,
  this chapter)

¼ cup softened butter *or*
  softened margarine

½ teaspoon vanilla extract

1 cup chopped walnuts *or*
  pecans (optional)

Place brown sugar, sugar, and cinnamon in a bowl. Mix well. Add flour and mix well. Add butter or margarine and vanilla, mixing until the topping is coarse and crumbly. Add nuts, if using, and mix in well.

This topping may be used instead of a top crust on a pie. It also works well when used on cakes; just sprinkle the topping on the batter before baking.

7

Monstrously Delicious Cookies and the World's Best Brownies

After much experimenting, we discovered that the new insulated double-layer "never burn" cookie sheets are well worth the money. If you don't have a set or don't want to spend the money, try using two regular cookie sheets, one right on top of the other. Because using alternative flours and ingredients results in cookie doughs that are not as "sticky" as those made from bleached, enriched flour made from wheat, our cookie doughs spread as they heat up; a regular cookie sheet tends to allow the dough to heat too rapidly and almost fry onto the sheet before it can bake.

Baking one sheet of cookies at a time, placed on the center rack of the oven, allows the heat to circulate more evenly in the oven. A slightly lower oven temperature allows the dough to bake thoroughly while lessening the chance of having edges or bottoms burn. Finally, chilling the dough by shoving the bowl right into the refrigerator before forming the batches of cookies, and allowing the cookie sheets to cool thoroughly before baking the next batch, may help keep the dough firmer while it bakes.

Cookie Flour Chart

These are suggested combinations of flours that work well for cookies. All combinations are for 1 cup flour.
NO means the flour alone or that combination of flours is not appropriate for a good cookie.
OK means the flour may be used by itself and does not require another flour in addition to it.
ANY COMB. means any ratio of the two flours that adds up to 1 cup will make a good cookie.

	Amaranth	Barley	Chickpea/Garbanzo	Millet
Amaranth	OK	¼ cup barley with ¾ cup amaranth	¼ cup chickpea with ¾ cup amaranth	up to ¼ cup millet with ¾ cup or more amaranth
Barley	¼ cup barley with ¾ cup amaranth	OK	¼ cup chickpea and ¼ cup barley with ½ cup quinoa, oat or spelt	up to ¼ cup millet and up to ¼ cup barley with ½ cup or more quinoa, oat or spelt
Chickpea/ Garbanzo	up to ¼ cup chickpea with ¾ cup or more amaranth	¼ cup chickpea and ¼ cup barley with ½ cup or more quinoa, oat or spelt	NO	up to ¼ cup chickpea and up to ¼ cup millet with ½ cup or more quinoa, oat or spelt
Millet	up to ¼ cup millet with ¾ cup or more amaranth	up to ¼ cup millet and up to ¼ cup barley with ½ cup or more quinoa, oat or spelt	up to ¼ cup millet and up to ¼ cup chickpea with ½ cup or more quinoa, oat or spelt	NO
Oat	ANY COMB.	¼ cup barley with ¾ cup oat	up to ¼ cup chickpea with ¾ cup or more oat	up to ¼ cup millet with ¾ cup or more oat

	Amaranth	Barley	Chickpea/Garbanzo	Millet
Quinoa	ANY COMB.	¼ cup barley with ¾ cup quinoa	up to ¼ cup chickpea with ¾ cup or more quinoa	up to ¼ cup millet with ¾ cup or more quinoa
Spelt	ANY COMB.	¼ cup barley with ¾ cup spelt	up to ¼ cup chickpea with ¾ cup or more spelt	up to ¼ cup millet with ¾ cup or more spelt

	Oat	Quinoa	Spelt
Amaranth	ANY COMB.	ANY COMB.	ANY COMB.
Barley	¼ cup barley with ¾ cup oat	¼ cup barley with ¾ cup quinoa	¼ cup barley with ¾ cup spelt
Chickpea/Garbanzo	up to ¼ cup chickpea with ¾ cup or more oat	up to ¼ cup chickpea with ¾ cup or more quinoa	up to ¼ cup chickpea with ¾ cup or more spelt
Millet	up to ¼ cup millet with ¾ cup or more oat	up to ¼ cup millet with ¾ cup or more quinoa	up to ¼ cup millet with ¾ cup or more spelt
Oat	OK	ANY COMB.	ANY COMB.
Quinoa	ANY COMB.	OK	ANY COMB.
Spelt	ANY COMB.	ANY COMB.	OK

Aaron's Honey-Barley Cookies

Makes 2 dozen cookies

½ cup honey
¹⁄₃ cup mild-tasting oil
1¼ cups barley flour
½ teaspoon baking powder
¼ teaspoon baking soda
¼ teaspoon salt
½ teaspoon vanilla extract

Preheat oven to 325°F. Grease cookie sheet.

In a large bowl, combine all ingredients and mix well. Drop the dough by teaspoonfuls onto greased cookie sheet. Bake for 12–15 minutes or until the cookies begin to turn golden brown. Cool on cookie sheet.

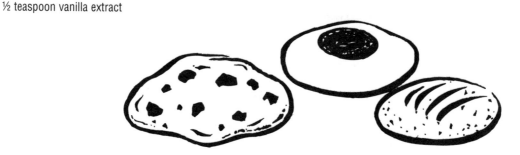

Bird's Nest Cookies

Makes 2 dozen cookies

½ cup softened margarine *or* softened butter

¼ cup light or dark brown sugar, packed

1 egg yolk

½ teaspoon almond extract

1 cup flour (e.g., ¾ cup oat *or* spelt and ¼ cup barley *or* millet; *or* see chart, this chapter)

1 cup finely chopped nuts (any type)

⅓ cup jam, jelly, *or* preserves, any flavor (see chapter 9 for recipes)

Preheat oven to 350°F. Lightly grease cookie sheet.

Cream the margarine or butter with the brown sugar, egg yolk, and almond extract until smooth and almost fluffy. Fold in the flour and mix well. Place the chopped nuts in a shallow bowl and set aside. Form the dough into small balls, approximately ½-inch in size, then roll each ball in the chopped nuts. Place the coated balls on the greased cookie sheet and bake for 7–8 minutes.

Remove the cookie sheet from the oven, and make a deep depression in the center of each cookie ball with your thumb or the tip of a spoon, being careful to not go all the way through the cookie to the sheet. Spoon a small amount of jam, jelly, or preserves into the depression and return the cookie sheet to the oven to bake for another 8 minutes.

Carrot Cookies

Makes 2 dozen cookies

1 cup flour (e.g., ¾ cup oat
  or spelt and ¼ cup barley *or*
  millet; *or* see chart, this
  chapter)

1 teaspoon baking powder

¼ teaspoon salt

½ cup sugar

2 egg yolks *or* ½ teaspoon
  Ener-G Egg Replacer powder

½ cup butter *or* margarine *or*
  mild-tasting oil

½ cup cooked and mashed
  carrots

Preheat oven to 400°F. Grease cookie sheet.

Combine the flour, baking powder, salt, and sugar. Add the egg yolks or Ener-G Egg Replacer powder, butter or margarine or oil, and carrots. Mix until well blended. Drop by teaspoonfuls onto greased cookie sheet.

Bake for 8 minutes. Cool cookies on cookie sheet.

Chocolate Drop Cookies

Makes 3 dozen cookies

½ cup sugar

¾ cup softened margarine *or* softened butter

1 egg yolk

1 teaspoon almond extract *or* vanilla extract

¼ cup carob powder *or* cocoa powder

1½ cups flour (e.g., ¾ cup oat and ¾ cup barley; *or* see chart, this chapter)

Preheat oven to 375°F. Use ungreased cookie sheet.

In a large bowl, beat the sugar, margarine or butter, egg yolk, and almond or vanilla extract until fluffy. Stir in the carob or cocoa powder and beat again until fluffy. Stir in the flour ½ cup at a time, mixing well after each addition. By teaspoonfuls, drop the dough onto the cookie sheet, leaving 1 inch between cookies.

Bake for 6–8 minutes. Using a spatula, place the cookies immediately on a platter for cooling.

Cinnamon Gobbles

Makes 2 dozen cookies

¹/₃ cup mild-tasting oil *or* softened margarine

¹/₃ cup maple syrup

¹/₃ cup yogurt (cow's milk *or* soy; plain, vanilla, *or* maple-flavored)

1 teaspoon baking soda

1 teaspoon cinnamon

¾ cup flour (such as oat *or* spelt; *or* see chart, this chapter)

Preheat oven to 350°F. Grease and flour cookie sheet.

Cream together the oil or margarine, maple syrup, and yogurt until smooth. Add the baking soda and cinnamon; beat well. Add the flour and beat until almost fluffy. Drop the batter by teaspoonfuls onto cookie sheets, leaving 2½ inches between cookies.

Bake for 10 minutes or until the cookie edges begin to turn golden. Cool on the cookie sheet, then place the cookies on a platter, carefully lifting each cookie with a spatula. You may also refrigerate them overnight for a firmer cookie.

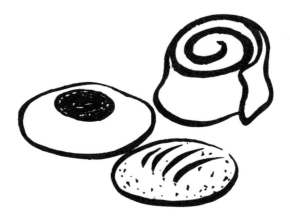

Gingersnaps

Makes 2 dozen cookies

¾ cup softened margarine *or* softened butter

1 cup sugar*

1 egg yolk

¼ cup light or dark brown sugar, packed

2 teaspoons baking soda

1 teaspoon each ground cloves, ginger, and cinnamon

¼ teaspoon salt

2½ cups flour (e.g., 1 cup oat, 1 cup spelt, and ½ cup barley; *or* see chart, this chapter)

*For a darker and richer taste, substitute ½ cup molasses for ½ cup of the sugar.

Preheat oven to 325°F. Use ungreased cookie sheet.

In a large bowl, cream the margarine or butter, sugar, egg yolk, and brown sugar together until fluffy. Add baking soda, cloves, ginger, cinnamon, and salt, beating again until fluffy. Add the flour, ½ cup at a time, mixing well after each addition. Drop the dough by generous teaspoonfuls onto the cookie sheet and very slightly flatten each cookie with the palm of your hand.

Bake 12–15 minutes or until the cookie edges become golden brown. Cool the cookies on the baking sheet.

Jacob's Drizzle Drop Cookies

Makes 3 dozen cookies

Cookie

½ cup sugar

1 pinch salt

½ cup softened margarine *or* softened butter

½ teaspoon vanilla extract

½ teaspoon almond extract

1 rounded teaspoon arrowroot flour mixed with ¼ cup water

1½ cups oat bran *or* quick oats

Drizzle Topping

¼ cup semisweet carob chips *or* chocolate chips

2 tablespoons margarine *or* butter

Preheat oven to 350°F. Grease cookie sheet.

For the cookies: Cream together all the cookie ingredients except the oat bran or oats. Once the dough is well blended and airy, stir in the oat bran or oats. Do not overmix. The dough is crumbly but will bake solid cookies. Drop the dough by teaspoonfuls onto the cookie sheet, leaving 2 inches between cookies. Bake 4–6 minutes or until the edges become golden brown. Once the edges have browned, remove the cookies from the oven and let them cool on the cookie sheet for 2 minutes, then place them on a large platter in a single layer.

For the topping: In a large saucepan, melt the carob or chocolate chips and the margarine or butter over low heat on top of the stove, stirring constantly. Once the chips are completely melted, drizzle the topping over the cooled cookies with a spoon. Refrigerate the cookies to set the chocolate drizzle topping.

Josh's Chocolate Chip Cookies

This rich and delicious cookie is perfection, not too cakey or too crisp.

Makes 3 dozen cookies

- 1 cup softened butter *or* softened margarine
- 1 teaspoon vanilla extract
- 1 cup light or dark brown sugar, packed
- 1 cup sugar
- 2 egg yolks *or* 3 teaspoons Ener-G Egg Replacer powder
- ½ teaspoon salt
- 1 teaspoon baking powder
- 2¼ cups flour (e.g., 1¼ cups oat, ½ cup barley, ½ cup spelt; *or* see chart, this chapter)
- 12 ounces carob chips *or* chocolate chips (mini-chips or regular size)

Preheat oven to 350°F. Use ungreased cookie sheet.

Cream together butter or margarine, vanilla, brown sugar, and sugar. Add egg yolks or Ener-G Egg Replacer powder and cream well. Add salt and baking powder; mix well. Add the flour, ½ cup at a time, mixing well after each addition. After all the flour is mixed in, stir in the chips.

Place one tablespoonful of dough in the palm of your hand and gently form a ball. Still using the palm of your hand, lightly press the dough onto the cookie sheet but do not flatten it! Leave approximately 2 inches between the balls of dough.

Bake for 11–12 minutes or until the cookies flatten somewhat and the edges begin to turn golden brown. Cool the cookies on the baking sheet; after they have cooled, use a spatula to move them to a plate.

Oatmeal Cookies

Makes 2 dozen cookies

¾ cup softened margarine *or* softened butter

¼ cup light or dark brown sugar, packed

1 egg yolk

⅓ cup cow's milk *or* soy milk *or* rice milk *or* almond milk

½ teaspoon vanilla extract

3 cups quick oats

1 cup flour (any one or combination of oat *or* spelt; *or* see chart, this chapter)

½ teaspoon baking soda

½ teaspoon salt

¼ teaspoon cinnamon

1 cup raisins (optional)

1 cup chopped nuts (optional)

Preheat oven to 375°F. Grease cookie sheet.

In a large bowl, cream margarine or butter, brown sugar, egg yolk, milk, and vanilla until fluffy. Add oats, flour, baking soda, salt, and cinnamon. Beat again until well mixed. Stir in raisins and nuts, if desired. Drop by tablespoonfuls onto cookie sheets and bake for 10–12 minutes or until cookies are lightly browned. Cool on cookie sheet.

Sugar Cookies

Makes 2 dozen cookies

½ cup softened margarine *or* softened butter

¾ cup sugar

1 tablespoon cow's milk *or* soy milk *or* rice milk *or* almond milk

1 egg yolk

½ teaspoon vanilla extract

¼ teaspoon salt

¼ teaspoon baking powder

1¼ cups flour (e.g., ½ cup oat, ½ cup barley, and ¼ cup soy; *or* see chart, this chapter)

Preheat oven to 375°F. Grease cookie sheet.

In a large bowl, cream margarine or butter, sugar, and milk. Beat in egg yolk and vanilla until fluffy. Add salt and baking powder, beating again until well mixed. Add flour, ½ cup at a time, and mix well after each addition. Chill the dough for 30 minutes or more in refrigerator. Drop the dough by tablespoonfuls onto the cookie sheet, leaving at least 2 inches between cookies. Bake for 7–9 minutes or until cookie edges begin to turn golden brown. Cool on cookie sheet.

The World's Best Brownies

This makes a very chocolaty, satisfying, and cakey brownie.

Makes 18 large brownies

1 cup mild-tasting oil *or* softened butter *or* softened margarine

2 cups sugar *or* 2 cups less 2 tablespoons honey

2 teaspoons vanilla extract

6 teaspoons Ener-G Egg Replacer powder

½ teaspoon baking powder

½ teaspoon salt

²/₃ cup cocoa powder

1¼ cups flour (e.g., ½ cup rice, ¼ cup buckwheat, and ½ cup spelt; *or* see chart, this chapter)

1 cup chopped walnuts (optional)

Preheat oven to 300°F. Grease two 8-inch square cake pans.

Beat the oil or butter or margarine with sugar or honey and vanilla until completely mixed. Add Ener-G Egg Replacer powder, baking powder, salt, and cocoa powder. Mix well. Add the flour and beat until completely mixed. Add nuts, if desired. Spread the batter into the pans.

Bake for 25 minutes or until the batter starts to pull away from the sides of the pans and an inserted toothpick comes out clean. Cool brownies in pan, slice, and serve.

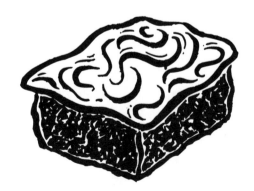

Toffee Squares

Some people say the molasses flavor in this dessert is too strong, but others like it. You decide.

4½ cups quick oats

¼ cup light or dark brown sugar, packed

¾ cup melted margarine *or* melted butter

½ cup sugar syrup* *or* ¼ cup dark molasses

1 tablespoon vanilla extract

½ teaspoon salt

12 ounces carob chips *or* chocolate chips

½ cup sliced almonds (optional)

---

*Note, to make sugar syrup heat ½ cup sugar and $^1/_8$ cup water together in a small saucepan over low heat until the sugar is completely dissolved and has just begun to caramelize.

Preheat oven to 400°F. Grease one 9" x 13" cake pan.

Mix the oats, brown sugar, margarine or butter, sugar syrup or molasses, vanilla, and salt very well. Press the mixture firmly into the baking pan. Bake for 15 minutes or until the mixture becomes bubbly. Remove the pan from the oven and turn the oven off. Immediately sprinkle carob or chocolate chips over the top and return the pan to the oven until the chips are completely melted (up to several minutes). After the chips have melted, remove the pan from the oven and cool for 10 minutes. Then sprinkle on the almonds and lightly press them into the carob or chocolate topping. Cool completely, cut into squares, and serve.

Tropical Fruit Bars

Makes 2 dozen bars

Filling

2 cups chopped dates

1 tablespoon vanilla extract

2½ cups canned unsweet-
ened crushed pineapple,
with juice

Base

1 cup oat flour

1 cup unsweetened shredded
coconut

½ cup chopped pecans *or*
walnuts

3 cups quick oats

¼ cup light or dark brown
sugar, packed

1 cup orange juice

¼ cup softened margarine *or*
softened butter *or* mild-tasting oil

Preheat oven to 350°F. Grease one 9" x 13" cake pan.

For the filling: In a medium saucepan, simmer the dates, vanilla, and pineapple until the mixture begins to thicken, stirring occasionally. Once it begins to thicken, remove the filling from the heat and set aside.

For the base: In a medium bowl, combine the flour, coconut, nuts, oats, and brown sugar; mix well. Add the orange juice and margarine or butter or oil; mix thoroughly. Press half of this base mixture into the cake pan. Pour all of the filling over this base evenly. Spread the remaining half of the base mixture evenly over the filling. Bake for 30–40 minutes, until the top crust is golden brown.

Cool in the pan and then slice into squares.

Doughnut Holes

Makes 2 dozen doughnut holes

3 cups oil (for frying)

4 cups flour (e.g., 3 cups oat *or* spelt and 1 cup barley *or* millet; *or* see chart, this chapter)

1 teaspoon salt

1 teaspoon any one or combination of nutmeg, cinnamon, and allspice

1 tablespoon baking powder, mixed with 3 tablespoons club soda

1 tablespoon honey

$\frac{1}{3}$ cup melted butter *or* melted margarine *or* mild-tasting oil

1 cup soy milk *or* rice milk *or* almond milk *or* water

In a deep fryer or saucepan, heat 3 cups oil.

In a large bowl, combine the flour, salt, and spices. Add the baking powder mixed with club soda, honey, butter or margarine or oil, and milk or water; mix until the dough is well blended and smooth.

Drop the dough by single teaspoonfuls into the deep fryer; fry until the doughnut holes are golden brown. Do not crowd them. Fry only a few at one time.

Remove the holes with a slotted metal spoon and drain on paper towels. Serve warm.

Energy Balls

These will last several weeks refrigerated.

Makes 2–3 dozen

½ cup Better Than Milk powder *or* goat's-milk powder *or* cow's milk powder, unreconstituted

½ cup granola (see chapter 9 for recipe)

½ cup oat bran

⅔ cup unsweetened coconut flakes or shredded coconut

1 cup nut butter (e.g., almond, peanut, *or* your choice)

½ cup honey

In a large bowl, combine the milk powder, granola, oat bran, and coconut. Mash in the nut butter and the honey until all ingredients are well mixed. Shape into 1-inch balls, place on a serving platter, cover, and chill for several hours before serving.

8 Special Desserts

Once in a while, the urge overwhelms you to create a sensational dessert that will knock your family's socks off. Turn to these recipes when winter chill begins creeping in the kitchen door, or when company is coming for Sunday dinner and it is too hot to bake a cake. No need to worry that your child will feel awkward or left out because he or she cannot share that special dessert; these are allergen-free and absolutely delicious!

Your choices range from custard to mousse to pudding. We also have a versatile shortbread that may be served as a dessert cookie or topped with fruit and used as a shortcake. Serve sherbet or sorbet for a cool ending to hot summer days, and our tapioca will warm anyone's heart any time of year.

We guarantee that at least one of these desserts will allow you to dance from the kitchen bearing a treat that will make their eyes light up and their lips go "Oooo!"

Sweet Potato Custard

*This dessert gets its mild sweetness from the sweet potatoes and juices—
there is no need for extra sugar.*

Makes 4–6 servings

2 cups cooked and mashed
sweet potatoes *or* yams

16 ounces medium or soft
tofu, drained and uncooked

3 tablespoons orange juice *or*
apple juice, undiluted

½ cup margarine *or* butter

5 egg yolks *or* 6 teaspoons
Ener-G Egg Replacer pow-
der mixed with 4 teaspoons
water

2 teaspoons grated lemon
peel

1 teaspoon cinnamon

½ teaspoon nutmeg

¼ teaspoon allspice

¼ teaspoon cloves

1 teaspoon vanilla extract*

½ cup cow's milk *or* soy milk
or rice milk

---

*Note: If you use vanilla-flavored soy
milk or rice milk, reduce the vanilla
extract to ½ teaspoon.

Preheat oven to 350°F. Use one ungreased 1½-quart casserole dish.

Combine all the ingredients in a blender or food processor and mix until the batter is completely smooth and free of lumps. Pour the batter into the baking or casserole dish and bake for 1 hour or until an inserted table knife comes out clean. Chill well before serving.

Quick Chocolate Mousse

Makes 2 servings

2 tablespoons strong coffee, almost boiling

¾ cup cow's milk *or* soy milk *or* almond milk, almost boiling

6 ounces carob chips *or* chocolate chips

3 tablespoons dark rum

1 egg yolk *or* ½ teaspoon Ener-G Egg Replacer powder mixed with ½ teaspoon water

Be sure the coffee and milk are hot to almost boiling; they must be hot enough to melt the carob or chocolate and cook the egg in order for the mousse to set well. Pour the coffee and milk into a blender. Add carob chips or chocolate chips and dark rum. Blend on the high setting for 3 seconds. Add the egg yolk or Ener-G Egg Replacer powder and blend on the high setting for another 2 minutes.

Pour the mousse into individual dessert dishes and chill for 6–8 hours.

Chocolate Marbled Pudding

Makes 4 servings

½ cup sugar

2½ tablespoons arrowroot flour

⅛ teaspoon salt

2 cups cow's milk *or* soy milk *or* almond milk

2 ounces unsweetened chocolate *or* carob, chopped coarse

3 egg yolks, beaten

2 ounces white chocolate, chopped fine

In a medium saucepan, combine sugar, arrowroot flour, salt, and milk; heat over medium heat, stirring until smooth. Reduce the heat to low and stir in the unsweetened chocolate or carob, stirring constantly until the chocolate or carob is melted and the pudding begins to thicken.

Remove the saucepan from the heat and slowly add the egg yolks, stirring constantly to prevent clotting. Return the saucepan to medium heat and stir for another 2 minutes.

Remove the saucepan from the heat, pour pudding into a medium size bowl and cover with plastic wrap; let the pudding cool for 5 minutes, then stir in the white chocolate just until it has blended in. Pour the pudding into a serving bowl or four individual dessert bowls. Serve warm, or let it cool in the refrigerator before serving.

Variation: You can cook this pudding in your microwave using a large microwave-safe bowl. Microwave it on HIGH for 2–4 minutes each time the recipe says to heat it on the stove, and remember to stir after each minute.

Brownie Pudding

Makes 4–6 servings

1 cup any flours containing gluten (e.g., ½ cup oat and ½ cup potato; or see chart, chapter 1)

½ cup sugar

6 tablespoons unsweetened carob powder or cocoa powder, divided

2 teaspoons baking powder

½ teaspoon salt

½ cup cow's milk or soy milk or rice milk or almond milk

2 tablespoons mild-tasting oil

1 teaspoon vanilla extract

½ cup finely chopped nuts (any type)

½ cup dark brown sugar, packed

¼ cup water

Preheat oven to 350°F. Lightly grease one 8-inch square baking pan.

In a medium bowl, combine the flour, sugar, 3 tablespoons of the carob or cocoa powder, baking powder, and salt and mix well. Add the milk, oil, and vanilla and beat until smooth. Fold in the nuts. Pour the batter into the baking pan.

In a separate small bowl, mix the brown sugar and remaining 3 tablespoons carob or cocoa powder, then sprinkle this over the batter in the baking pan. In a small saucepan, heat the water just until hot and pour it over the batter in the baking pan.

Bake for 45 minutes or until the pudding top begins to get crusty and the bottom layer begins to thicken. Serve warm or cool.

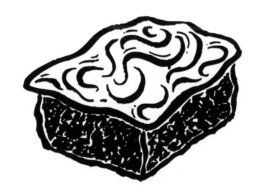

Fruit Sherbet

Makes 2–4 servings

1 tablespoon unflavored gelatin

¼ cup cold water

2 cups fruit juice (any type)

1 cup chopped fruit (any type)

In a freezer-safe mixing bowl, dissolve the gelatin in the cold water, stirring to dissolve it completely. Add the fruit juice and chopped fruit. Place the bowl in the freezer and leave it until the mixture is "mushy" ice, testing every 20 minutes or so. Once the mixture has become mushy, remove the bowl from the freezer and beat the sherbet until fluffy. Return the bowl to the freezer and freeze until solid, usually overnight.

Shortbread

This works very well for strawberry shortcake when you use brown sugar.

Makes one 8-inch square or 9-inch round shortbread

1 cup softened margarine *or* softened butter *or* mild-tasting oil

¼ cup sugar *or* dark or light brown sugar, packed

½ teaspoon vanilla extract

2 cups flour (e.g., 1 cup oat, ½ cup barley, and ½ cup millet; *or* see chart; chapter 1)

Preheat oven to 300°F. Use one ungreased 8-inch cake pan or one ungreased 9-inch springform pan.

Cream together the margarine or butter or oil, sugar or brown sugar, and vanilla very well. Slowly blend in the flour, ½ cup at a time, mixing well after each addition. Press the dough evenly into the cake pan; then, using the back of a fork, press the tines around the edges of the dough to make a scored pattern, and press the points of the tines all over the surface of the dough to make a dotted pattern.

Bake 45–50 minutes or until the center is almost firm to the touch and the surface has become a light golden color. Remove the shortbread from the oven and, leaving it in the baking pan, slice it immediately into wedges or squares. Cool and serve.

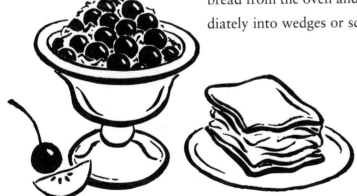

Raspberry Sorbet

Makes 4–6 servings

1¾ cups water
1¾ cups sugar
3 tablespoons lemon juice
½ tablespoon creme de cassis (black currant liqueur)
3 pints raspberries, rinsed

In a medium saucepan, combine the water and sugar. Bring to a boil to dissolve sugar completely, stirring frequently. Boil for an additional 2 minutes. Remove the saucepan from the heat and stir in the lemon juice and creme de cassis. Pour into a large bowl and let cool completely.

In a blender or food processor, puree the raspberries and strain them through a fine wire mesh strainer to remove all the seeds, then pour the pureed raspberries into the cooled sorbet. Refrigerate until completely chilled (several hours). Pour the chilled sorbet into a shallow baking pan or several ice cube trays and freeze until almost solid. Break the sorbet into chunks (or remove cubes from trays) and puree again in a blender or food processor.

Pour the sorbet into a freezer-safe bowl or container and freeze it for at least 1 hour before serving. Sorbet should be served fairly solid, but not completely frozen.

Tapioca

Makes 2–4 servings

2 cups water *or* any type fruit juice

3 tablespoons pearled tapioca

1 teaspoon vanilla extract

In a large saucepan, bring the water or juice to a boil. Stir in the tapioca pearls and let the mixture come to a boil again, then immediately remove the saucepan from the heat. Let the tapioca sit, covered, for 3 minutes. Return the saucepan to the stove, uncover, and bring the tapioca to a boil again, allowing the mixture to boil for 5 minutes, stirring two or three times a minute. Remove the saucepan from the heat and stir in the vanilla.

Pour the tapioca into a serving bowl and chill it in the refrigerator before serving.

9 Breakfast Ideas

Are you used to grabbing the variety cereal boxes at the store? Has breakfast always meant frying up some eggs and bacon or tossing sliced bread into the toaster and grabbing the butter and grape jelly? Get ready for some new ideas! Even grownups will enjoy these breakfast treats: some familiar old favorites, like pancakes and muffins, some new mouth-awakening flavors, like granola and apricot jam. Use these recipes as the groundwork for setting a whole new breakfast table, changing and adding ideas and ingredients of your own as you go along.

Pancakes and waffles are a wonderful and filling breakfast. Pancakes are ready to be turned over in the frying pan when the shine starts to disappear from the top of the batter and tiny bubbles begin to appear around the edges. Flip them once and cook for the same amount of time on the other side. You will get a feel for knowing when they have cooked all the way through after you make a few batches.

For homemade jams, jellies, and preserves, test for doneness by dripping a small amount of the jam or jelly, while it is simmering, onto a spoon and placing the spoon in the freezer for five minutes. Touch it and taste it. It should be thick but not hard, and just sweet enough. If it seems thin or runny, cook or microwave the jam for another five minutes, then retest.

Buckwheat Pancakes

*Makes 8–10 pancakes or
2–3 large waffles*

1 cup oatmeal

½ cup buckwheat flour

¼ teaspoon salt (optional)

1 teaspoon baking powder

¼ cup water *or* cow's milk *or* soy milk *or* rice milk

1 tablespoon butter *or* margarine *or* mild-tasting oil

1 teaspoon honey

Place the oatmeal in a blender and mix on high until ground into a course flour.

In a medium bowl, mix all ingredients until well blended and almost all the lumps are gone. Let the batter sit for several minutes to thicken; then stir vigorously by hand for several minutes more.

Pour the desired amount of batter for each pancake into a pre-heated oiled or buttered frying pan or waffle iron. Cook until bubbles appear around the edges of each pancake. Turn and cook for the same amount of time on the other side. Serve hot.

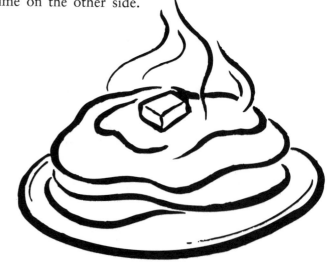

Mary's Pancake and Waffle Mix

This recipe is very lightly spiced and aromatic when cooking and is much less expensive than the ready-to-use wheat-free mixes.

Makes 3 cups of mix

1 cup oat flour
1 cup buckwheat flour
1 cup spelt flour
¼ teaspoon each cinnamon, nutmeg, and allspice
3 teaspoons baking powder
5 teaspoons Ener-G Egg Replacer powder

Combine all ingredients well. This mix can be stored in an airtight jar or container for up to 4 months.

To make 10 pancakes or 3 large waffles: In a medium bowl beat 1 cup of mix with ¾ cup any liquid (water, cow's milk, soy milk, rice milk, or almond milk). If you make a big batch of pancakes or waffles, you can store them in the freezer. They will heat up very well in your toaster whenever you want pancakes or waffles but have no time to make them from scratch.

Breakfast Muffins

*Makes 12 large or
24 regular muffins*

2 cups oat bran *or* 1 cup oat flour and 1 cup spelt flour

¼ cup light or dark brown sugar, packed

2 teaspoons baking powder

½ teaspoon salt

3 teaspoons Ener-G Egg Replacer powder

1 cup cow's milk *or* soy milk *or* goat's milk *or* almond milk

¼ cup honey

2 tablespoons butter *or* margarine *or* mild-tasting oil

½–1 cup fresh or frozen cranberries (to taste)

1 small banana, mashed

Preheat oven to 400°F. Line cupcake tin with cupcake papers.

Combine the oat bran or flours, brown sugar, baking powder, salt, and Ener-G Egg Replacer powder well. Add the milk, honey, and butter or margarine or oil and mix well. Add the cranberries and banana, mixing only until fruit is blended into the batter. If the batter feels too stiff, add a little more milk by teaspoonfuls until the desired consistency is reached. Fill the cupcake papers two-thirds full.

Bake for 15 minutes or until tops of muffins are lightly browned and an inserted toothpick comes out clean. May be served warm or stored in the refrigerator or freezer and microwaved on HIGH for 30 seconds to reheat.

Variation: Instead of the cranberries and bananas, try one of the following:

½ cup finely chopped apple, with 1 teaspoon ginger, cinnamon, or allspice

1 cup pitted cherries or blueberries

½ cup canned crushed pineapple drained with ½ teaspoon grated orange peel

½ cup finely chopped nuts (any type)

Buckwheat Muffins

*Makes 10 large or
15 regular muffins*

¾ cup buckwheat flour

¾ cup any other flours (e.g.,
¼ cup soy *or* rice and ½
cup millet *or* oat)

2 teaspoons baking powder

½ teaspoon salt

1 cup water *or* cow's milk *or*
soy milk *or* rice milk

5 tablespoons honey

¼ cup mild-tasting oil

2 egg yolks *or* 3 teaspoons
Ener-G Egg Replacer pow-
der mixed with 2 teaspoons
water

1 teaspoon vanilla extract

½ cup raisins (optional)

½ cup sunflower seeds
(optional)

Preheat oven to 350°F. Line cupcake tin with cupcake papers.

In a large bowl, mix together the flours, baking powder, and salt. Add the water or milk, honey, oil, egg yolks or Ener-G Egg Replacer mixture, and vanilla; beat until smooth. Add raisins and seeds, if desired, and mix until well blended. Fill the cupcake papers two-thirds full.

Bake for 20 minutes or until tops of muffins are lightly browned and an inserted toothpick comes out clean.

Sweet Granola

This recipe has been modified to use flax oil, which contains an essential fatty acid shown to be helpful with skin problems and middle ear infections. However, any mild-tasting oil, margarine, or butter can be used and the results are always delicious!

Makes approximately 7 cups of granola

½ cup flax oil *or* any mild-tasting oil *or* melted butter *or* melted margarine

½ cup honey *or* maple syrup

½ cup light or dark brown sugar, packed

1 teaspoon vanilla extract

4 cups rolled oats (regular, instant, or "quick")

1 cup cashews *or* almonds, slivered, sliced, or pieces (but not crushed)

½ cup flax seeds *or* sunflower seeds (optional)

1 cup chopped dates

1 cup raisins

Preheat oven to 300°F. Use one ungreased cookie sheet.

Mix the oil or butter or margarine with the honey or maple syrup, brown sugar, and vanilla. Add the rolled oats, nuts, seeds, dates, and raisins; mix well. Spread the granola evenly onto the cookie sheet and bake for 20 minutes. Remove the sheet from the oven and turn the granola over completely; then bake for another 10 minutes. Remove the granola from the oven and stir well. Let it cool completely before storing.

The granola will keep well in a large jar in the cupboard or a covered bowl in the refrigerator for several weeks.

Apricot Spread

Makes 16 ounces

8 ounces dried apricots
¾ cup water
¼ cup honey
1 tablespoon orange juice
¼ teaspoon cinnamon
2 8-ounce jars

In a large saucepan, heat the apricots and water over a high heat until boiling. Reduce the heat and simmer for 15 minutes or until the apricots are very tender. Remove the saucepan from the heat, let sit for about 10 minutes, and then pour off the excess water. Stir in the honey, orange juice, and cinnamon. Pour the spread into a blender or food processor and blend until almost smooth. Pour the spread into the jars. The apricot spread will keep up to two months stored in the refrigerator.

Honey-Orange Syrup

Makes 8 ounces

¾ cup honey

1 teaspoon butter *or* margarine

1 tablespoon grated orange peel

¼ cup orange juice

1 teaspoon orange extract

1 8-ounce jar

In a medium saucepan, heat the honey and butter or margarine over medium heat until bubbling. Remove the saucepan from the heat and stir in the orange peel, juice, and extract, mixing well. Pour the syrup into a jar. It will keep up to one month stored in the refrigerator. Reheat before serving if desired.

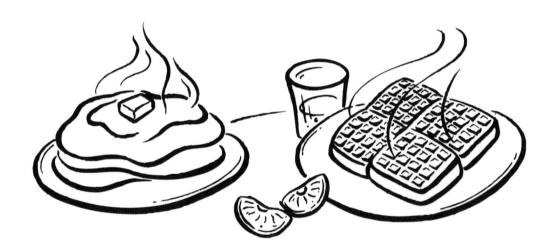

Old-Fashioned Minty Jam

Makes 30 ounces

1 pound (3 large) nectarines *or* peaches, pitted and chopped

½ cup orange juice concentrate, undiluted

1 pint blueberries *or* boysenberries, rinsed

10 fresh mint leaves, minced fine

4 8-ounce canning jars with new lids and rings

In a large nonaluminum saucepan, heat the nectarines or peaches and orange juice over a medium heat until the mixture begins to simmer. Continue simmering for 5–7 minutes, stirring occasionally. Stir in the blueberries or boysenberries and continue simmering for another 3–5 minutes, until jam begins to thicken. Remove the saucepan from the heat and add the mint, stirring well. Spoon the jam into 8-ounce canning jars; clean any drips from the mouths of the jars and screw on the lids, making sure the rings are tight.

To seal the jars, fill a large, deep pot with enough water to submerge the jars 1 inch below the water surface. Bring the water to a boil. Using tongs, place the filled jars in the boiling water, and boil for 10 minutes. Remove the jars with tongs and let them cool to room temperature.

Store the jam in the cupboard or the refrigerator. It will keep up to one year if the jar is not opened or one month after opening if kept in the refrigerator.

Microwave Apricot Jam

Dried apples or peaches may be used instead of apricots, and apple juice may be used instead of orange juice, for different lovely flavors.

Makes 40 ounces

16 ounces dried apricots
2½ cups orange juice
¾ cup sugar
½ teaspoon cinnamon
¼ teaspoon ground ginger
1 tablespoon lemon juice
3 16-ounce jars

In a large microwave-safe bowl, combine the apricots, orange juice, and sugar. Cover loosely and microwave on HIGH for 12 minutes. Pour the mixture into a blender or food processor. Add the cinnamon, ginger, and lemon juice; blend until smooth. Pour the jam into the jars. It will keep up to two months stored in the refrigerator.

Microwave Cherry Preserves

Makes 40 ounces

36 ounces fresh or frozen dark cherries, pitted

½ cup sugar

½ tablespoon lemon juice

3 16-ounce jars

In a large microwave-safe bowl, combine the cherries and the sugar. Cover loosely and microwave on HIGH for 12 minutes. Remove and stir to completely dissolve the sugar; leave uncovered and microwave on HIGH for another 40–45 minutes. Pour the mixture into a blender or food processor, add the lemon juice, and blend until the cherries are coarsely pureed. Pour into the jars. It will keep up to two months stored in the refrigerator.

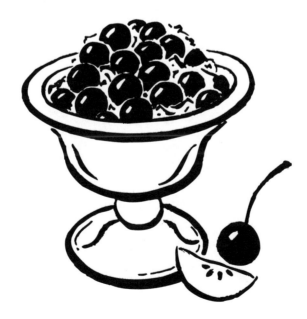

Microwave Fresh Peach Jam

Makes 8 ounces

1½ cups (2 medium) peach-
es, peeled and chopped

4 tablespoons sugar

1 tablespoon arrowroot flour

¼ teaspoon ground ginger

¼ teaspoon allspice

1 teaspoon lemon juice

1 8-ounce jar

In a 1½-quart microwave-safe casserole dish, combine all ingredients except the lemon juice. Microwave, uncovered, on HIGH for 4 minutes. Stir the jam well, then microwave, uncovered, for an additional 3–4 minutes or until the jam begins to thicken. Using a fork, mash any large chunks of peaches. Stir in the lemon juice and set the jam aside to cool until it is lukewarm. Once it is cooled, cover the bowl or spoon the jam into the jar and refrigerate overnight before using. The jam will keep up to one month stored in the refrigerator.

Microwave Strawberry Jam

Makes 32 ounces

3 pints fresh strawberries, washed, hulled, and halved

1½ cups sugar

1 tablespoon lemon juice

2 16-ounce jars

In a 2½ quart microwave-safe bowl, combine the strawberries, sugar, and lemon juice. Cover loosely and microwave on HIGH for 15 minutes. Stir the jam to completely dissolve the sugar; leave uncovered and microwave for another 40–45 minutes. Spoon the jam into jars and refrigerate overnight before using. The jam will keep up to two months stored in the refrigerator.

Berry Smoothie

Makes 1 serving

1 ripe banana, chilled and peeled

½ cup strawberries, chilled and hulled

¼ cup dates, pitted

1 tablespoon bee pollen (optional)

3 tablespoons honey

1 cup cold fruit juice (any type)

½ cup crushed ice or 3 small ice cubes

In a blender, puree the banana, strawberries, and dates until smooth. Add the bee pollen, if using, and honey, blending until smooth. Add the fruit juice and ice and blend on high speed until smooth. Serve immediately.

Tropical Smoothie

Makes 1 serving

¼ cup orange juice

¼ cup pineapple juice

1 tablespoon coconut milk

½ banana, peeled

¼ teaspoon fresh peeled and
grated ginger

½ cup crushed ice or 3 small
ice cubes

Place all ingredients in a blender and mix on high until well blended. Serve immediately.

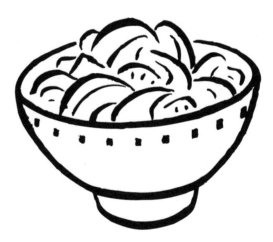

Fruit Smoothie

Makes 6 servings

1 very ripe cantaloupe,
  peeled, seeded, and diced

2 tablespoons frozen orange,
  lemonade, *or* limeade concentrate, undiluted

1 tablespoon honey

¼ teaspoon cinnamon

¼ teaspoon cardamom

1 liter unflavored seltzer
  water

In a blender, puree the cantaloupe until smooth. Add the frozen juice, honey, cinnamon, and cardamom; blend until smooth. Chill in a container for several hours. To serve, mix equal amounts of the smoothie with the seltzer water.

Power Smoothie

Makes 1 serving

¼ cup oat bran flakes

⅓ cup cold water

8 ounces lemon yogurt, dairy or nondairy

1 cup fresh or frozen berries (any kind)

½ teaspoon grated lemon peel

In a blender, mix the bran flakes on high speed until almost powdered. Add the cold water and let sit for several minutes. Add the yogurt, berries, and lemon peel and blend on high speed until smooth. Serve immediately.

10 Can I Still Shop at My Local Supermarket?

*T*his chapter does not endorse any products, nor is it a complete list of all available food products. It merely lists foods we now commonly purchase that are readily available at most local grocery stores, along with ingredient information that we have discovered by trial and error.

Your child may have an allergy to a food that is not addressed in this book, such as gluten. You will have to use the list of gluten flours in chapter 1 to help you eliminate gluten products from your child's diet, and also go to other sources for help in creating gluten-free meals. For any allergy you are coping with, your first source of information is your eyes: Be sure to read all ingredient lists carefully. Many ingredients are commonly known in the food industry under several different names. Ask your doctor for help with other possible names for the ingredients your child is allergic to. Call a manufacturer's toll-free phone number and request specific information about labeling and ingredient sources.

Also, remember that many children's medicines have a corn-based sweetener added to make them more palatable, and many children's vitamins have a corn-based sweetener and/or cornstarch added for taste and stability. Ask your doctor to verify the ingredients in any medication, and ask your pharmacist for labeling information on vitamins.

The following gives names these foods are frequently identified as:

Corn: Bran, caramel, cerelose, dextrose, fructose, germ meal, glucose, gluten meal, grits, hominy, HVP (hydrolyzed vegetable protein), Karo, maize, maltodextrin, masa harina, modified food starch, polenta, pozole, sucrose, and xanthan gum.

Cow's milk: Casein, curd, lactalbumin, lactoglobulin, lactose, sodium caseinate, rennet, whey. (Note: Calcium carbonate and calcium lactate are *not* dairy-derived ingredients.)

Egg: Albumin, "ovo."

Wheat: Accent, bran, bread crumbs, bulgur or burghol, couscous, cracker meal, durum, farina, many forms of "filler," gluten, graham, HVP (hydrolyzed vegetable protein), many types of modified food starch, MSG, orzo, Postum, pumpernickel, seitan, semolina, tabbouleh, some varieties of tempeh, wheat germ, and some forms of yeast.

Now that you have plowed through this list and are quaking at the thought of spending the next three days reading supermarket labels just to be able to get dinner on the table, don't give up. It is time-consuming and frightening at first, but we promise it will get easier. And you will also receive the best reward possible—a healthy, happy child. Finally, remember that fresh fruits and vegetables are a great snack.

This list describes common ingredients and the additions frequently associated with them:

Baking powder Most commercial baking powders have cornstarch added to insure a free-pouring, lump-free product. Plain baking soda is sometimes an acceptable alternative (see chapter 2), and cornstarch-free baking powders (also called cereal-free), such as Featherweight, are available at most health food stores.

Catsup The only commercial brand we found that was free of corn syrup sweetener was a kosher catsup carried during the Jewish holidays. All other catsups had corn syrup sweetener, and many also contained artificial ingredients.

Cereals Plain oatmeals, most instant oatmeals, Rice Chex, and puffed rice cereals are all corn- and wheat-free.

Chocolate candy Many confectioners' boxed chocolates, such as Fanny May or Fannie Farmer, have an egg white gloss brushed onto the candies for consumer eye appeal. Plain chocolate bars, such as Hershey's, do not have the egg white gloss; but remember that most milk chocolate bars use a cow's-milk derivative, and their ingredients must be checked carefully. Also, "white" chocolate is derived from the cacao bean, and its use should be OK'd by your doctor if your child has a chocolate allergy.

Cocoa Cocoa powder and chocolate powder usually have cornstarch added to insure a dry, lump-free, and free-flowing product; if specific ingredient information is not available on the label, play it safe and melt baker's chocolate for your baking needs. Carob powder and carob chips are wonderful "chocolaty" alternatives if you are dealing with a chocolate allergy, but you must also check their labels for corn and cow's-milk additives.

Confectioners' sugar or powdered sugar Most confectioners' or powdered sugar has cornstarch added to ensure a dry and free-flowing product. You can make a reasonable substitute by slowly pouring small amounts of granulated sugar into your food processor or blender while it is on high speed (see chapter 2 for recipe). This will not give you as fine a powder, but it still works well.

Cookies Almost all cookies use wheat flour and some sort of corn sweetener, a lot use butter or some form of cow's-milk products, and a few use eggs. We have not found any allergen-free supermarket cookies; however, health food stores and many mail-order companies offer a variety of acceptable packaged cookies. Check the labels for ingredients appropriate to your child. We have found the labeling to be very specific and quite useful. HeavenScent and Nature's Warehouse cookies are tasty and reasonably priced.

Crackers Rice crackers now come in lots of different flavors. These are healthy and crunchy alternatives to potato chips, popcorn, and other snacks popular with kids. Several varieties of RyKrisp are also wheat- and corn-free, and many supermarkets and restaurants have these available.

Fruit Roll-Ups or fruit leathers Some commercial fruit roll-ups do not contain corn syrup sweeteners. You may object, however, to the amounts of artificial coloring and flavoring they use. Health food stores usually have organic fruit roll-ups or leathers (dried, pressed fruits), such as Stretch Island Fruit Leather manufactured by Stretch Island Fruit, Incorporated, Grapeview, Washington. You may want to check for nitrates used in the drying process, which may concern you as it does us.

Gelatin Several brands of boxed gelatin mixes are corn-free; however, many use Nutrasweet, which may concern you as it does us.

Ice cream Some ice creams, such as Breyer's Chocolate and Breyer's Mint Chocolate Chip, do not contain eggs, egg whites, or corn syrup sweeteners. However, all ice creams, ice milks, sherbets, and frozen yogurts are made from cow's milk. Most health food stores and many local supermarkets now carry frozen tofu desserts, which are delightful alternatives. Many health food stores also have frozen rice milk "ice creams" such as Rice Dream, which are delicious.

Juice Many brands of frozen and fresh fruit juices are made from juice and water only, but check labels carefully for any corn-based sweeteners. At restaurants, an assurance that orange or grapefruit juice is freshly squeezed should be sufficient.

Malt Most malts are derived from barley and are acceptable as nonallergic products. Malt also provides additional minerals and vitamins when mixed with cow's milk, rice milk, or soy milk.

Margarine We found only two brands of margarine in our local supermarket that were corn- and dairy-free: Parkay Squeeze Spread in a plastic bottle and a generic store brand of spread in a large plastic tub at Jewel Food Stores. Your supermarket may offer its own generic brand, but be sure to check the label for acceptable vegetable-based ingredients. Since most people with an allergy to cow's milk are reacting either to the whey or to the casein, check with your allergist to find out if either is acceptable in your child's diet.

Mayonnaise All commercial brands of mayonnaise contain egg; some contain corn oil. Use an egg-free, corn oil-free salad dressing instead.

Milk We have found soy milk and goat's milk readily available at our local supermarkets. Powdered goat's milk, tofu drinks, and rice and almond milks can be found at health food stores.

Molasses Commercial brands of light and dark molasses, which are used in many baked goods such as gingersnap cookies, are acceptable and do not contain corn products.

Mustard Many contain wheat flour as a thickener; find a brand that clearly states all its ingredients.

Oils Many oils at your supermarket are clearly labeled and contain only one type of pure oil, such as canola or olive. However, carefully check the bottles marked "vegetable oil" as they may contain corn oil.

Potato chips Some brands of potato chips are deep-fried in oils other than corn oil. A rigorous label search may reward you. Caution: Labels reading "all vegetable oil" may mean corn oil or peanut oil is used with other oils. If the list of ingredients is not specific and your store manager or the manufacturer cannot supply the information, play it safe and avoid the product.

Puddings Several brands of ready-to-eat pudding cups are wheat- and egg-free. For example, Del Monte uses corn and tapioca as the bases for their modified food starch, and beet sugar or cane sugar as the bases for their sweetener. However, remember that unless otherwise specified these products contain cow's milk.

Rice Many brands of rice are "enriched"—the nutritious hull has been stripped off, vitamins and minerals have been artificially added to the kernels, and the final product has been dusted with cornstarch to keep the grains loose and dry. Always buy a brand that is "converted": the kernels have been pressure-cooked to drive the nutrients from the hull into the grain, and the kernels do not need to be kept dry artificially; it is also a more nutritious product.

Salt Most brands of iodized table salt contain dextrose as a stabilizing ingredient, and many of those brands also contain sodium silicoaluminate, an aluminum by-product, which may concern you as it does us. However, many grocery stores also carry sea salt and "pickling" or "preserving" salts. These function just as well as iodized table salt for cooking and baking, and are dextrose- and sodium silicoaluminate-free. Some manufacturers offer iodine-free table and cooking salts that do not contain dextrose. If you are concerned about a lack of iodine in your child's diet and the possible impact on their thyroid, discuss this with your doctor or licensed nutritionist, and consider adding sea salt to your pantry and table. Other good sources of iodine include shellfish, saltwater fish, dried seaweed, cod liver oil, and vegetables grown very near an ocean. Also, please remember that kosher or "sour" salt is not an acceptable substitute for table salt or for baking desserts.

Sorghum A sweetener derived from a domestic grain, sorghum is acceptable and does not contain corn products. However, it has a very strong taste that some people dislike.

Soy sauce Most brands of soy sauce use wheat in the distillation process. Carefully check labels to obtain an acceptable soy sauce, or buy tamari, which is usually made without wheat.

Vanilla Many brands of vanilla extract, imitation vanilla flavoring, and other types of extracts and flavorings use grain alcohol as the base in the extraction process. It is usually a wheat-based alcohol. Most also list "corn syrup sweetener" or "dextrose" as additional ingredients. If your local store does not carry an acceptable vanilla, a specialty or gourmet food store or health food store will usually have one, or you may try making your own (see chapter 2 for recipe).

Vinegar White (clear) vinegars are distilled from a variety of grains, fruits, and vegetables, while cider (brown) vinegar normally uses apple cider as its base. Since cider vinegar usually has as high a level of acidity (the important factor in baking, cooking, and pickling) as white vinegar, people with grain and potato allergies may use cider vinegar with confidence.

Yogurt Yogurt is almost always a cow's-milk product. Some stores now carry a creamy yogurt-like tofu, a soy product, or a goat's-milk yogurt. These are tasty alternatives, all of which are available flavored with fruits.

11 Green Cleaning and Safe Pesticides

*K*eeping our homes clean is almost a full-time job in itself. Since you already spend time cleaning, and now are even more concerned because your child's allergies may include pollen, spores, and dust mites, why not simply use "earth-friendly" cleaning products and botanical, or plant-derived, pesticides instead of pouring more chemicals around? This chapter begins with cleaning tips, continues with gardening tips, and ends with a list of botanical suppliers and brochures for more detailed information. Insecticide and pesticide suppliers and your local nursery are usually more than happy to discuss your particular gardening or insect problem. Just be careful about using any chemicals. Just because a sales clerk assures you that minimal use is fine doesn't mean it is fine. The Center for Pest Control in Washington, D.C., has some wonderful people to help you, and they can send pamphlets pertaining to your needs. GreenPeace also has some free helpful literature about ecologically safe cleaning supplies and alternatives to commercial products.

HOUSEHOLD CLEANERS

Baking soda A wonderful alternative to chlorine powders and liquids. Baking soda and vinegar can be used to "boil" out mineral deposits in glasses and pots and pans and to eliminate calcified areas on the tub and bathroom sink (with a little elbow grease). If you use baking soda boxes as a deodorant in the freezer or refrigerator, once the recommended three months is up you may still use the baking soda as a cleaning product.

Dishwasher detergent A more chemical-free detergent can be made by combining a commercial detergent with equal amounts of powdered borax and washing soda (2 cups commercial detergent plus 2 cups borax plus 2 cups washing soda). GreenPeace recommends eliminating the commercial detergents entirely, but I have found that a film similar to hard-water spots coats my dishes and glasses when I don't use any commercial detergent, so I cheat and add it.

Flax soap A good alternative to commercial linoleum cleansers, although you will have to rinse carefully to get rid of the dull effect it may leave on no-wax floors. It is also wonderful for washing any wood in your house, including floors, furniture, and kitchen cabinets. Most furniture made since World War I is sealed at the factory with long-lasting impenetrable lacquers, and the wood underneath does not need to be "nourished" by oils or waxes; it can be cleaned and treated well simply by using ¼ cup flax soap to one gallon of water and washed with a clean sponge or rag.

Vinegar A good alternative to commercial cleansers and to ammonia when cleaning windows and leather desktops. It also works for dusting: combine 2 tablespoons white vinegar in 1 quart warm water, pour into a spray bottle, and spray onto a clean cloth for dusting and cleaning leather, or directly onto mirrors or windows for streak-free cleaning.

INDOOR PEST CONTROL

Ants Powdered boric acid is an effective ant control. Take a jar lid, spoon in a little jam, jelly, or honey, sprinkle generously with powdered boric acid, and leave it where you have noticed ants. They will climb in to eat the sweets, ingest the boric acid, and trail it home to the ant colony. Within a week the colony will be all or mostly all dead. Please keep boric acid away from carpets and furniture as it has a corrosive effect on these materials. Please also keep it away from children and pets: it is harmful in large enough doses.

Tannic acid, an ingredient in caffeinated teas, is also a good insecticide. In a large nonaluminum pot, boil 1 gallon of water with 12–16 teabags, then let it steep until the water is almost black. Remove the teabags and pour the tea around the outside of your home, paying special attention to areas where you think ants have built their colonies. It may take several gallons over a week or two, but the ants will diminish or disappear.

Cockroaches Many people have found that sprinkling powdered boric acid in cupboards and along baseboards helps to control cockroaches. Whole bay leaves placed in drawers and cupboards also seems to be a fairly effective control; fresh bay leaves work better and faster than dried bay leaves, but dried ones will eventually work.

Dust mites These tiny insects live in carpeting, furniture, mattresses, pillows, stuffed animals, and just about anything people can own. Vacuuming and mopping alone will not eliminate them. Allergy Control Products, Incorporated, sells a spray that kills dust mites and is nontoxic to people and animals. See chapter 12 for their address.

Fleas Brewer's yeast and/or a garlic supplement added to your dog's or cat's food will help control fleas and is undetectable to the animals as they eat. For dogs, try using 1 scant tablespoon of brewer's yeast every other day, and/or 1 garlic tablet weekly, ground and mixed into your pet's food (you may have to increase the dosage if you see no effect in a week). For cats, try using 1 scant teaspoon of brewer's yeast every other day, and/or 1 small garlic tablet weekly. If you don't have garlic tablets, finely chop 1 small clove. A tiny amount of eucalyptus oil spread carefully on the dog's or cat's collar will also help control fleas, but don't use so much that it can seep into the pet's skin or rub off where the pet can lick it—even botanical solutions can be deadly to a small animal. If available, use eucalyptus leaves or lemon gum (*Eucalyptus citriodora*) to make a "pillow" for the pet's bed; it is not as effective as quickly, but certainly safer. Ecologically safe pyrethrin sprays, available at your local gardening center or by mail order (see chapter 11) can be used directly on animals (check the label or with your veterinarian for correct amounts). Please note that citrus solutions are toxic to pets, whether as a dip or as a wipe. Cedar chips and shavings, spread in the pet's pen or made into a pillow for the pet's bed, are definitely safe and do work—cedar is registered with the Environmental Protection Agency as a flea repellent. But please check with your veterinarian before using any form of insecticide.

Household plant insects and mites A simple rinsing of the plant leaves in cool water in your sink every two to three weeks will eliminate most pests from indoor plants.

OUTDOOR PEST CONTROL

Always test the spray or powder on one or two leaves first to determine the plant's sensitivity. If the leaves are OK after several days, you may use the spray or powder on the whole plant.

Fungicides Mix 1 teaspoon organic insecticidal soap with 3–4 teaspoons baking soda, 3–4 teaspoons vegetable oil, and 1 gallon tap water. Pour into spray bottles and spray all leaves on both sides several times a week for one week.

Insect control with sprays and powders Safer's Soap, available at most commercial garden centers and nurseries or by mail order from most gardening supply catalogs, is an effective pest control. Follow the container instructions for use. Or you can make your own outdoor garden pest control liquid by using one of the following recipes:

1. Mix 1 tablespoon liquid dish soap (not detergent) with 1 cup vegetable oil; add 1–2 teaspoons of this mixture to 1 cup tap water, pour into a spray bottle, and spray your plant leaves and fruits.

2. Put 3–4 garlic cloves in the blender with 1 cup tap water. Blend until liquefied, pour the mixture into a spray bottle, and spray your plant leaves and fruits.

3. Make your own pyrethrin spray by purchasing pyrethrin concentrate from your local nursery and following the directions on the container; or grow and pluck *Chrysanthemum cinerariifolium* flower heads when two or three outer rows of petals have opened in the central yellow discs. Dry the flower heads either in sunlight or in your oven set on the lowest temperature. Grind the heads into a powder using a coffee mill, blender, or mortar and pestle. Pour 10 grams of the powder into a dark-colored bottle (light will weaken the solution) and add 4 ounces of denatured alcohol; shake and let stand for 24 hours at room temperature. Pour into a spray bottle and spray directly onto affected plants. Pyrethrin kills insects and fish on contact, but is considered safe in very small amounts when it comes into surface contact with humans and other warm-blooded animals.

4. Diatomaceous earth (a finely ground powder made from the fossilized remains of primitive plants known as diatoms) sprinkled in your garden area will kill exoskeletar (chitinous, or with the skeleton on the outside) insects. The sharp edges of these microscopi-

cally small ground plants pierce the insect's shell, allowing its vital fluids to leak out. Please be careful when spreading diatomaceous earth, because it should not be breathed in; use a mask and scatter carefully when there is no wind.

All these mixtures break down after exposure to sunlight and moisture, and will rinse off with rain and dew. They are not recommended for indoor plant use. You must be careful using any type of pest control, indoors or outside.

Beneficial insects May easily be used to control outdoor pests. Ladybugs will attack aphids; green lacewings will eat aphids, mealy grubs, whiteflies, mites, and thrips' eggs and larvae; spined soldier bugs will eat large caterpillars; and praying mantises will help control a variety of pesky insects. Beneficial insects and their proper care and usage can be ordered from any of the suppliers listed at the end of this chapter.

Companion plantings If you want to avoid pests in the garden without resorting to chemical sprays or lots of work, try companion planting. Grow insect-repelling flowers and herbs in your garden, such as marigolds and nasturtiums to keep out beetles, whiteflies, and nematodes; and spearmint to keep ants at bay; geraniums to repel Japanese beetles; garlic and chives to help fight aphids, Japanese beetles, and weevils; rosemary to make life miserable for cabbage moths; borage to keep hornworms from chewing up your tomatoes; and tansy or pennyroyal as a general all-around repellant. Other types of flowers attract birds, which eat insects. Since some plants seem to be natural bug repellants and other plants seem to attract bugs, interplanting the repellants between the rows of vegetables and herbs that attract nuisance bugs will work as a fairly effective and natural pesticide. For example, pennyroyal (*Mentha pulegium*) is a form of common mint with a very strong, almost resinous, aroma and a large amount of naturally occurring pulegone, a toxic insect-repelling compound.

If you don't know which plants to use, contact your local nursery or one of the several resources at the end of this chapter.

Mosquito repellent To repel mosquitoes, take 500–1,000 units of vitamin B1 orally ½ to 1 hour before going out. It lasts for several hours.

ECOLOGICAL CLEANING RESOURCES

Arm & Hammer Use Wheel Offer (cleaning booklet using baking soda)
PO Box 7285
Monticello, MN 55563-7285
$1.00 booklet (make check payable to Church & Dwight Company, Incorporated)

Annie Berthold-Bond, *Clean and Green: The Complete Guide to Nontoxic and Environmentally Safe Housekeeping*
Ceres Press
Paperback, $8.95
Ask your local bookseller to order a copy if none is available or check your local library.

Beverly De Julio (environmentally safe cleaning booklet)
PO Box 111
Palatine, IL 60078
Free.

GreenPeace (cleaning and pesticide information poster)
1436 U Street N.W.
Washington, D.C. 20009
(202) 462-1177
Price information is unavailable. Often GreenPeace gives free information booklets when you make a donation. They have also been an invaluable resource over the phone.

Mothers and Others (annual newsletter, cleaning information, and alternatives booklet)
40 W. 20th Street
New York, NY 10011
(212) 242-0010
$25.00 annual tax-deductible contribution for all of the above.

3M Company (safer furniture stripping and refinishing products; filters for furnaces and air conditioners)

3M Center
Consumer Relations
Bldg. 515-3N-02
Maplewood, MN 55144-1000
(800) 364-3577

May be purchased at your local hardware store, or call 3M's consumer relations telephone number, above, for more information.

20 Mule Team Borax (free cleaning booklet using borax)

Dial Corporation - CIC
15101 N. Scottsdale Road–MS 5028
Scottsdale, AZ 85254
(800) 528-0849

ORGANIC HERBICIDE AND PESTICIDE SUPPLIERS AND ORGANIZATIONS

Arbigo (for organic pesticides and other supplies)

PO Box 4247
Tucson, AZ 85738
(800) 827-2847

Beneficial Insectary (beneficial insects)

14751 Oak Run Road
Oak Run, CA 96069
(916) 472-3715

BioLogic (beneficial insects)

PO Box 177
18056 Springtown Road
Willow Hill, PA 17271
(717) 349-2922

Bozeman Bio-Tech (organic pesticides and other supplies)

1612 Gold Avenue
Bozeman, MT 59715
(800) 289-6656
Free catalog.

Companion Plants (botanical pesticide controls)
7247 N. Coolville Ridge Road
Athens, OH 45701
(614) 592-4643
Catalog $2.00.

Eco Safe Products (organic pesticides)
PO Box 1177
St. Augustine, FL 32085
(800) 274-7387

Gardener's Supply (beneficial insects)
128 Intervale Road
Burlington, VT 05401
(802) 863-1700

Gardens Alive! (beneficial insects and Sunspray UltraFine Spray Oil)
5100 Schenley Place
Lawrenceburg, IN 47025
(812) 537-8650

Garden Ville (beneficial insects and other supplies)
6266 Highway 290 West
Austin, TX 78735
(512) 892-0006

National Center for Environmental Health Strategies
1100 Rural Avenue
Voorhees, NJ 08043
(609) 429-5358
Contact for information.

National Coalition Against the Misuse of Pesticides
701 East Street S.E., Suite 200
Washington, D.C. 20003
(202) 543-5450
Contact for information.

Nature's Control (beneficial insects)

PO Box 35
Medford, OR 97501
(503) 899-8318

Stoller Enterprises, Incorporated (for Golden Natur'l Spray Oil)

8585 Katy Freeway
Houston, TX 77024
(281) 461-1493

W. Atlee Burpee Company (beneficial insects and other gardening supplies)

300 Park Avenue
Warminster, PA 18974
(800) 888-1447

12 Resources

Many cities and towns do not have conveniently located health food stores, and your local supermarket may not carry grains, flours, or other baking ingredients suitable for your child. We have contacted each of the manufacturers and sellers listed here to verify that they will ship to individuals or to buying clubs. Most of the catalogs are free; some cost a minimal amount. All will charge shipping and handling costs. Buying in bulk, however, will limit the money you have to spend on those charges. We store our grains and flours in airtight plastic containers or glass jars, which eliminate any possible bug problem and allow us to purchase and store much more than just one pound at a time. Just remember to label your containers immediately. Many of the gluten and nongluten flours look very similar to one another. Also, if you feel you will not use up the flours within two months, store them in airtight containers in the freezer to prevent souring. Already-baked breads are best stored in the freezer immediately after purchasing them.

You might also want to check with your accountant or tax preparer to see if any of the special ingredients, foods, and allergy products you must now buy for your allergic child, and any of the attendant costs such as specialty cookbooks and shipping charges are tax deductible as medical expenses. A general rule of thumb is that if your doctor has prescribed special products, including foods, for your allergic child because of an elimination diet, you may deduct the cost of the foods that exceeds the cost of the nonallergic foods; for example, if your doctor has prescribed wheat- and corn-free products and a loaf of white bread is available at the supermarket for $.89 and a loaf of spelt bread the same size costs $3.50, you may deduct $2.61, the difference between what you would have paid for the white bread and what you must now pay for the spelt bread.

Manufacturers and suppliers are listed alphabetically, followed by allergy control products, allergy and asthma support organizations, and cookbooks we found helpful.

INGREDIENTS MANUFACTURERS AND SUPPLIERS

Aphrodisia

282 Bleecker Street

New York, NY 10014

(212) 989-6440

Nonorganic herbs, baking powders, and some other baking ingredients.

Free catalog; will ship small orders to individuals. UPS shipping charge and $4.00 handling charge will be added.

Arrowhead Mills, Incorporated

PO Box 2059

Hereford, TX 79045-2059

(800) 858-4308

Grains, beans, seeds, nut and seed butters, oils, breakfast cereals, flours, and ready-to-make mixes.

Call for a list of retailers in your area. Arrowhead Mills does not sell to individual consumers.

Dietary Specialties

PO Box 227

Rochester, NY 14601

(800) 544-0099

Cake and bread mixes, cookies, crackers, cereals, gluten-free products, pastas, flours, and baking products.

Free catalog. Payment may be made by check, money order, or credit card. Shipping and handling charges begin at $4.20.

Eden Foods, Incorporated

701 Tecumseh Road

Clinton, MI 49236

(313) 973-9400 or (517) 456-7424

EdenSoy soy-milk products, grains, and canned goods. Call for a list of retailers in your area. Eden Foods does not sell to individual consumers.

Ener-G Foods, Incorporated

PO Box 84487

Seattle, WA 98124-5787

(800) 331-5222

Ener-G Egg Replacer powder, flours, grains, breads, mixes, ready-to-make foods, recipes, pastas, nondairy beverages, and low-protein and gluten-free products.
Free catalog. Payment may be made by check, money order, or credit card. Shipping and handling charges begin at $4.00.

FoodCare, Incorporated

PO Box 6383

Champaign, IL 61821

(217) 687-5115

Alternative dairy products, breads, snacks and dried fruits, cereals, flours and grains, baking supplies, and convenience food products.
Free catalog. Payment may be made by check, money order, or credit card. UPS shipping and handling charges begin at $3.95.

Gold Mine Natural Foods

PO Box 3608

Chico, CA 95927

(800) 475-3663

Certified organic and kosher products, grains and beans, snacks, flours, household and personal products.
Free catalog. Payment may be made by check or credit card. UPS shipping and handling charges begin at $4.50 per order.

Grainaissance, Incorporated

1580 62nd Street

Emeryville, CA 94608

(510) 547-7256

Organic kosher plain and flavored rice milks, rice pudding, ready-to-bake rice doughs.
Call or write for ordering instructions.

Health Valley Foods, Incorporated

16100 Foothill Boulevard

Irwindale, CA 91706-7811

(818) 334-3241 or (800) 423-4846

Soups, pastas, prepared foods, soy milk, cookies and crackers, cereals.
Call for a list of retailers in your area. Health Valley Foods does not sell to individual consumers.

Indian River Organics

Box 12411-0

Fort Pierce, FL 34979

(407) 465-6652

Certified organic citrus fruits and vegetables.
Free brochure.

Jackson Mitchell

Meyenberg Goat Milk Products

PO Box 5425

Santa Barbara, CA 93150

Goat's-milk products and recipes.
Write for a list of retailers in your area. Meyenberg does not sell to individual consumers.

Jaffe Bros. Incorporated

PO Box 636

Valley Center, CA 92082-0636

(616) 749-1133

Organic dried fruits, nuts and butters, beans, grains, flours, and pastas.

Free catalog. Will ship small orders to individuals. Payment may be made by check, credit card, or C.O.D. Shipping and handling charges depend on weight of order. Will ship UPS or U.S. postal service.

The King Arthur Flour Baker's Catalogue

PO Box 876

Norwich, VT 05005-0876

(800) 827-6836

Flours, flakes, grains, baking tools and supplies, and dried fruits.

Free catalog. Payment may be made by check or credit card. Shipping and handling charges depend on weight of order. Will ship UPS or U.S. postal service.

Living Farms

PO Box 50

Tracy, MN 56175

(507) 629-4431

Certified organic whole grains and seeds.

Free catalog. Will ship small orders to individuals. Prepayment and UPS shipping charges may be paid by personal check.

Mountain Ark Trader

PO Box 3170

Fayetteville, AR 72702

(800) 643-8909

Large variety of food and baking products and ingredients.

Free catalog. Will ship any size order to individuals; rush delivery available. Payment and shipping charges may be paid by check, credit card, or C.O.D.

Natural Lifestyle Supplies

16 Lookout Drive

Asheville, NC 28804-3330

(800) 752-2775

Flours, grains, baking ingredients, cereals, beans, seeds, pastas, herbs, seasonings, sea salts, rice and soy milks, household and personal items.

Catalog $1.00. Will ship any size order to individuals; shipment via UPS or U.S. postal service. Costs vary by weight of order. Payment and shipping charges may be paid by check, credit card, or C.O.D.

North Farm Cooperative

204 Regas Road

Madison, WI 53714

(800) 236-5880

Grains, flours, ready-to-make foods and mixes, cereals, baking products and ingredients, frozen foods, canned goods, and household products.

Will ship to buying clubs in Wisconsin, Michigan, Illinois, Minnesota, Indiana, and parts of Missouri, Iowa, Ohio, Wyoming, South Dakota, North Dakota, and Montana. Call for catalog and details.

Nu-World Amaranth, Incorporated

PO Box 2202

Naperville, IL 60567

(630) 369-6819

All organic amaranth products, flours, and grains.

Free catalog. Will ship any size order via U.S. postal service or UPS. Costs vary by weight of order. Payment and shipping charges may be paid by check or money order.

Tad Enterprises

9356 Pleasant

Tinley Park, IL 60477

(708) 429-2101

All gluten-free products: flours, ready-to-make mixes, cereals, crackers and cookies, baking ingredients, and ready-to-eat products.

Free catalog. Payment may be made by check, money order, or C.O.D. Shipping and handling charges begin at $4.20.

Timber Creek Farms

PO Box 606

Yorkville, IL 60560-0606

(630) 553-1119

Certified organic produce, juices, meats, grains, nuts, and some flours.

Free catalog. Will ship small orders to individuals. UPS shipping costs start at $6.95; payment may be made by check or credit card.

Walnut Acres

PO Box 8

Penns Creek, PA 17862

(800) 433-3998

Large variety of certified organic whole grains, flours, and other foods.

Free catalog. Will ship any size order to individuals. Payment may be made by credit card, check, or money order. Shipping and handling charges start at $4.50 for UPS or U.S. postal service.

Wild River

PO Box 1711

Grass Valley, CA 95945

(916) 273-2661

Cereals, granola, soups, pasta, flours, and other food items.
Free catalog. Will ship any size order to individuals. Payment may
be made by credit card, check, or money order; UPS shipping
charges apply. Will ship C.O.D.

ALLERGY CONTROL PRODUCTS

Allergy Control Products, Incorporated

96 Danbury Road

Ridgefield, CT 06877

(800) 422-DUST

Mattress covers, pillowcases, blankets, room air cleaners, carpet
sprays, furnace filters, respiratory care products, allergy books and
cookbooks.
Free catalog. Payment may be made by credit card or check.

ORGANIZATIONS

American Academy of Allergy and Immunology

611 E. Wells Street

Milwaukee, WI 53202

(414) 272-6071

Provides information about allergies. Call for availability and
prices of tapes and brochures.

American College of Allergy and Immunology

800 E. Northwest Highway, Suite 1080

Palatine, IL 60067

(800) 842-7777

Medical facility that provides information about allergies and asth-
ma. Call for availability and prices of brochures.

American Dietetic Association's Consumer Nutrition Hotline

(800) 366-1655

For answers to your food and nutrition questions or for a referral to a registered dietitian in your area. Hotline operates 10:00 A.M. –5:00 P.M. E.T.

American Lung Association

1740 Broadway

New York, NY 10019

See your phone book or doctor for nearest chapter.

Ask-A-Nurse

(800) 535-1111

Free 24-hour phone service sponsored by local hospitals and staffed by registered nurses. Available in 38 states to answer general health questions. Call the above number to find out if the service is available in your area.

Asthma and Allergy Foundation of America

1717 Massachusetts Avenue

Washington, D.C. 20036

(800) 7-ASTHMA or (202) 265-0626

Provides information about asthma and allergies. Call for availability and prices of brochures.

Celiac Sprue Association (national headquarters)

PO Box 31700

Omaha, NE 68131-0700

(402) 558-0600

Food Allergy News

c/o The Food Allergy Network

4744 Holly Avenue

Fairfax, VA 22030-5647

(800) 929-4040

Bimonthly 8-page newsletter with recipes, dietitian's column, product updates, allergy research, and medication information; $18.00 annual fee.

Gluten Intolerance Group of North America

PO Box 23053

Seattle, WA 98102-0353

(206) 325-6980

National Allergy and Asthma Network/Mothers of Asthmatics

10875 Main Street, Suite 210

Fairfax, VA 22030

(800) 878-4403 or (703) 385-4403

Nonprofit group that provides information packets and books on asthma and videos for children ages 3–7. Call for availability and prices of brochures.

National Center for Nutrition and Dietetics

216 W. Jackson Boulevard

Chicago, IL 60606

(800) 366-1655

Nonprofit group that provides registered dietitians to answer diet and health questions Monday through Friday, 9:00 A.M.–4:00 P.M. CST.

National Jewish Center for Immunology and Respiratory Medicine

1400 Jackson Street

Denver, CO 80206

(800) 222-LUNG

Medical lung diseases facility that provides literature on asthma and other respiratory illnesses. Call for availability and prices of brochures.

COOKBOOKS

Baking for Health, Linda Edwards, Avery Publishing Group, Incorporated, $8.95.

Cooking for the Allergic Child, Judy Moyer, Grove Printing, $19.95. Available from Allergy Control Products, Incorporated, (800) 422-DUST. Call for additional shipping and handling costs.

More from the Gluten-Free Gourmet, Bette Hagman, Henry Holt, $25.00.

Quaker Oat Bran Favorite Recipes, created and published by The Quaker Oats Company, $3.50. To order call (800) 367-6287.

Appendix I

Common, Scientific, and Family Names

Common Name	Scientific Name	Family Name
Amaranth	*Amaranthus*	*Amaranthaceae*; Amaranth family
Arrowroot	*Maranta arundinacea*	*Marantaceae*; Arrowroot family
Barley	*Hordeum*	*Poaceae*; Grass family
Buckwheat	*Fagopyrum esculentum*	*Polygonaceae*; Buckwheat family
Chickpea/Garbanzo	*Cicer arietinum*	*Fabaceae*; Bean family
Kamut	*Triticum*	*Poaceae*; Grass family
Millet	*Pennisetum americanum*	*Poaceae*; Grass family
Oat	*Avena satica*	*Poaceae*; Grass family
Potato	*Solanum tuberosum*	*Solanaceae*; Potato family
Quinoa	*Chenopodium quinoa*	*Chenopodiaceae*; Goosefoot family
Rice	*Oryza sativa*	*Poaceae*; Grass family
Rye	*Secale cereale*	*Poaceae*; Grass family
Soy	*Glycine max*	*Fabaceae*; Bean family
Spelt	*Triticum aestivum*	*Poaceae*; Grass family
Teff	*Eragrostis ref*	*Poaceae*; Grass family
Wheat	*Triticum*	*Poaceae*; Grass family

By international convention, the scientific name of a species or genus is always set in italics.

REFERENCES

The Plant Book, D. J. Mabberly, Cambridge University Press, 1987.
Flowering Plants of the World, edited by V.H. Heywood, Mayflower Books.

Appendix courtesy of Dr. David G. Fisher.

Appendix II

FOOD FAMILIES

A food family is a botanical classification of foods that are related first by the flower structure and second by the genetic structure. A person with an allergy to one member of a specific food family may also be allergic to other foods in the same family. If your child is allergic to one food in a particular family, check with your doctor before using other members of that food family. Following is a list of food family names with the fruits, vegetables, nuts or grains which belong in that family listed below. This is not a complete list; however, it does reflect most of the ingredients used in this cookbook.

Agar family
  yeast
Amaranth family
  amaranth
Amaryllis family
  aquamil
Apple family
  apples (including cider and
    vinegar)
  pears
  quinces
Arrowroot family
  arrowroot
Banana family
  bananas

plantains
Bean or legume family
  carob
  chickpeas or garbanzo
    beans
  kudzu
  licorice
  peanuts
  soy (including soy flour,
    soy sauce, and tofu)
Birch family
  filberts
  hazelnuts
Buckwheat family
  buckwheat

rhubarb
sorrel
Cashew family
  cashews
  mangoes
  pistachios
Citrus family
  grapefruit
  lemons
  limes
  oranges
  tangerines
Composite family
  safflower
  sunflower

vermouth
Ginger family
  cardamom
  ginger
  turmeric
Gooseberry family
  currants
  gooseberries
Goosefoot family
  beets (and beet sugar)
  quinoa
Grape family
  cream of tartar
  grapes (including brandy,
    raisins, some vinegars,
    and some wines)
Grass family
  barley (and barley malt)
  cane sugar (and molasses)
  corn
  kamut
  millet
  oat
  rice
  rye
  spelt
  teff
  wheat
Heather family
  blueberries
  cranberries
  huckleberries
  wintergreen
Laurel family

cinnamon
sassafras
Honey family
  honey
Madder family
  coffee
Macadamia family
  macadamias
Maple family
  maple (including maple
    sugar and syrup)
Mulberry family
  breadfruit
  figs
  mulberries
Myrtle family
  allspice
  cloves
Nutmeg family
  mace
  nutmeg
Olive family
  olives (including green and
    black olives and olive oil)
Orchid family
  vanilla
Palm family
  coconuts
  dates
Pineapple family
  pineapple
Plum family
  almonds
  apricots

cherries
nectarines
peaches
plums (including prunes)
Potato family
  white potato
Rose family
  blackberries
  boysenberries
  loganberries
  raspberries
  strawberries
Sesame family
  sesame (including seeds
    and oil)
Spurge family
  tapioca
Sterculia family
  cocoa
  cola
Sweet potato family
  sweet potato
Walnut family
  black walnuts
  English walnuts
  hickory nuts
  pecans

Dr. Mandell's Allergy-Free Cookbook, Fran Gare Mandell, 1981.

The Allergy Survival Guide and Cookbook: To Your Good Health! Carolyn Stone and Jan Beima, 1988.

Index